Cooking with Rabbit

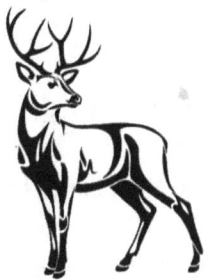

Laura Vosika

Gabriel's Horn Publishing

Copyright 2024 by Laura Vosika and Gabriel's Horn Press

All rights reserved. No portion of this book may be reproduced, stored in any retrieval system, or transmitted in any form or by any means electronic, mechanical, photocopy, recording, scanning, or other except for brief quotations in reviews or articles, without the prior written permission of the author and publisher.

Cover Design: Laura Vosika

Contact editors@gabrielshornpress.com

Published in the United States by Gabriel's Horn Press

First printing: 2024 Printed in the United States.
For sales, please visit www.gabrielshornpress.com
PRINT ISBN: 979-8-88846-089-4

Other Books by Laura & Chris

The Blue Bells Chronicles: a tale of time travel....
- *Blue Bells of Scotland*
- *The Minstrel Boy*
- *The Water is Wide*
- *Westering Home*
- *The Battle is O'er*

Food and Feast in the World of the Blue Bells Chronicles: a gastronomic historic poetic musical romp in thyme

The Four Spheres: habits for a better life

Go Home and Practice: a record book for music students and musicians for better progress

Gabriel's Horn Poetry Anthologies, collator/editor
- *Startled by JOY: 2019*
- *Startled by NATURE: 2020*
- *Startled by LOVE: 2021*
- *Startled by HUMOR: 2022*
- *Startled by MUSIC: 2023*
- *Startled by FAITH: 2024*

221 BC Dr. Kendall Price and Laura Vosika

Glenmirril Garden: original music in the style of Celtic jigs and reels; Laura Vosika with Judd Knauss

Things Beyond Our World: Stories of the Supernatural, Laura Vosika and Chris Powell

The Saint in the Cellar, by Laura Vosika and Chris Powell

On Wings of Light and Love: poetry and essays on love, Laura Vosika and Chris Powell

The Path that Shines: a story of life, love, and loss, by Chris Powell

COOKING

WITH

RABBIT

Table of Contents

Cooking with Rabbit

- Other Books by Laura & Chris 3
- Table of Contents 7
- INTRODUCTION 11
- MODERN RECIPES 15
  - BRAISED 17
    - Porcini Braised Rabbit 18
    - Braised Rabbit Pappardelle 19
    - Braised Rabbit with Tarragon, Mustard, and Cream 20
    - Cider Braised Rabbit 21
    - Rabbit Cacciotore (Italian, Braised) 22
  - FRIED 23
    - Shawn's Fried Rabbit 24
    - Korean Extra Crispy Fried Rabbit 25
    - Buttermilk Fried Rabbit 26
    - Mom's Fried Rabbit & Gravy 27
  - GRILLED 29
    - Mustard and Bacon Grilled Rabbit 30
    - Grilled and Marinated Garlic Rabbit 31
    - BBQ Grilled Rabbit with Mashed Potatoes 32
  - PORCHETTA 33
    - Rabbit Porchetta 34
    - Porchetta #2 35
    - Substituting Rabbit for Pork 38
    - Italian Pork Porchetta 39
  - ROASTED & BAKED 41
    - Roasted Rabbit in Wine Sauce and Garlic 42
    - Roasted Rabbit with Olive and Feta 43
    - Baked Rabbit & Chorizo Rice 44
    - Baked Rabbit with Apple and Lemon 45
    - Baked Rabbit in Mustard Sauce 46
  - STEWS 47
    - Rabbit and Dumplings 48
    - German Rabbit Stew 50
    - Slow-Cooked Rabbit Stew 52
    - Ischian Rabbit Stew, Italian 53
    - Greek Rabbit Stew (Rabbit Stifado) 54
    - Old Fashioned Rabbit Stew 56
    - Rabbit Stew with Mushrooms 58
    - Crock Pot Rabbit Chili 60

    White Rabbit Chili...61
STUFFED...63
    Rabbit Saddle with Ham and Mushrooms..64
    Stuffed Rabbit Roulade with Boudin..66
    Stuffed Rabbit with Chorizo and Scallops...68
    Stuffed Rabbit with Mushrooms, Spinach, and Cheese......................................70
PASTA..71
    Pulled Rabbit and Morel Ravioli...72
    Confit of Rabbit and Green Olive in Saffron Tortellini..74
    Rabbit Meatballs with Porcini Tagliatelle...77
    Rabbit Agnolotti Pasta..78
    Rabbit Ragu..80
    Tagliatelle with Rabbit in Mustard Sauce...81
TERRINES...83
    Rabbit and Pork Terrine with Peppercorns...84
    Olive and Pistachio Rabbit Terrine...86
    Rabbit Terrine with Bacon, Lemon and Herbs..88
PIES, CASSEROLES..91
    Rabbit Pie...92
    Old English Rabbit Pie...94
    Rabbit Casserole...96
SAUSAGE, MEATBALLS, MEATLOAF...97
    Making Rabbit Sausage...98
    Rabbit-Apple Sausage...101
    Rabbit Sausage with Fennel, Chili Flakes and Broccoli Rabe...........................102
    Parmesan Rabbit Sausage..103
    Rabbit Sausage with Garlic and Sweet White Wine..104
    Rabbit Meatloaf with Pepper Jack Cheese..105
    Rabbit Meatballs..106
MUFFINS, MISCELLANEOUS...107
    Muffins with Rabbit Meat and Cheese...108
    Rabbit and Gorgonzola Tart...109
    Orange Rabbit with Thermomix...110
    Sous Vide...111
    Fried Rabbit Sous Vide..112
    Rabbit Organ Meat Saute with Garlic Cream Bone Broth Sauce......................114
VARIOUS COUNTRIES...115
    Rabbit Curry—Indian..116
    Rabbit in Mustard Sauce — French...117
    Civet of Hare or Jugged Hare—French..118
    Sichuan Rabbit with Peanuts — Chinese..121
    Spicy Cold Rabbit Meat – Chinese..122
    Sweet and Sour Rabbit – Asian style...123
    Rabbit Ragu with Prosciutto—Italian...124

- Calabrian Rabbit with Red Peppers 126
- Belgian Rabbit Legs 127
- Hungarian Rabbit Paprikash 128

MEDIEVAL RECIPES 131
- Rabbit—Then and Now 132
- Rabbit in Gravy—Coneys in Gravy 133
- Rabbit in Wine Currant Sauce 134
- Rabbit in Broth—Connynges in grauey 135
- Medieval Rabbit 15th Century—Czech 136
- Medieval Rabbit Stew with Spices Civé de connin 138
- Rabbit in Wine or Ale Sauce 140
- Rabbit with Figs and Mudéjar Spices 141

NOTES 143
- Combinations 145
- Other Recipes 151
  - My Recipe: 152
  - My Recipe:: 153
  - My Recipe:: 154
  - My Recipe:: 155
  - My Recipe:: 156
  - My Recipe:: 157
  - My Recipe:: 158
- THANK YOU! 159

INTRODUCTION

Rabbit meat is not common fare in the United States. So why a cook book solely on rabbit meat? At Glenmirril Farms, we breed New Zealand White rabbits—for selling, for meat and for fur. When we began the switch from our suburban lives to more self-sufficiency, we started with growing plants. When I saw I could keep a head of lettuce alive, I made the bold move up to chickens. Our first four, Rhode Island Reds, were fantastic layers.

We wanted a source of meat in addition to chicken. I wasn't ready to jump all the way to cattle. We looked at goats and rabbits. My research showed me that rabbit meat is one of the healthiest meats there is. As a vital bonus, in my book (not this literal cookbook but my figurative book), nobody has ever been head-butted by or accidentally trampled to death by a rabbit—short of the Monty Python rabbit, but I'm pretty sure that's pure fiction. (Having a bunch of rabbits that look just like it, I hope so, at least.) We hadn't yet gotten fencing up for goats and this city girl felt safer with a twelve-pound rabbit than a twelve-hundred-pound cow. So, we got rabbits.

We chose New Zealand Whites because they're among the most common breed raised for meat rabbits—plus they're really beautiful.

WHY RABBIT:

In America, we no longer eat much rabbit. But we should. It's one of the healthiest, leanest, low-calorie meats you can eat. Compared to veal, beef, lamb, pork, turkey, or chicken, rabbit has the highest protein, lowest fat, and fewest calories per pound. It's low in cholesterol and fat; high in vitamin B, potassium, calcium, and phosphorous. It's good for the metabolism and great for cardiovascular health, or, in plain English, the heart

As per the old joke, the meat tastes a little like chicken…but with a somewhat stronger, meatier flavor. It can be prepared in virtually any way you'd prepare chicken: sautéed in oil or butter, fried, baked, breaded, braised, boiled, roasted, stuffed. One classic that is different from any chicken recipe I've ever seen is *lapin à la moutarde*: rabbit in mustard sauce.

In many parts of the world and in the past, eating rabbit was common. But it isn't today and hence, you won't find recipes for rabbit in the average cookbook. I had no recipes in my cookbooks to prepare our own rabbits. So I made one devoted to rabbits. My expectation was that, rabbit meat being an uncommon dish in the United States, I'd have to hunt long and hard for recipes. I found the opposite: I was so inundated by them, the trick was keeping the book short enough, as I intended it as an introduction to cooking with rabbit meat rather than a comprehensive source.

As a result, I've tried to include a variety of ways rabbit meat can be prepared: Stews, braised, baked, broiled, in casseroles, stews, pastas, chili, and with dumplings; as a main dish, with everything from mushrooms to red peppers, and even in tarts! Perhaps the only exception is ice cream. I haven't found a recipe for rabbit meat ice cream! Or a cocktail. I haven't come across a rabbit meat cocktail. If you find either of these, please let me know! Or maybe I'll make one just to prove a point.

I've included a variety of cuisines—Asian, Italian, Indian, French, Hungarian, and German to name a few. I've included recipes with a variety of flavors and spices and a section on medieval recipes with rabbit as it was more commonly used then—and in fact regarded as a dish for kings.

I encourage you to use this book as a start to exploring the many ways of cooking rabbit, and then seek out the wealth of recipes online. I encourage you to mix and match the recipes in this book: for instance, use the spices and seasonings from a baked recipe with braising or add the spices from an Italian recipe to a stuffed rabbit recipe.

If you find and prepare one you like, please let us know at: www.facebook.com/GlenmirrilFarms. We would love to have you post any pictures of the meals you make with rabbit meat and recipes.

HARE VS RABBIT

Hare and rabbits are related, but different animals. Hares are bigger and faster, have longer ears and haven't been domesticated. For the purpose of a cookbook, however, we don't really care how fast either can run, except of course if you're trying to catch one by chasing it. Then you might want to go for rabbit and hope for the best. I'd still bet on the rabbit. Nothing personal.

For cooking, the question is really about the difference in meat, however. Both can be eaten. Hare meat is said to be even healthier than rabbit meat, with lower fat and better lipid indices. Their meat is dark or red, with a strong gamey flavor. Rabbits, by contrast, are mostly white meat with a finer texture, more like chicken. Hare must be cooked longer than rabbit. This gives you time to rest up from what is likely to be a longer chase. The downside of course, is that unless you're an excellent shot and have a place to hunt, you may be hard-pressed to find hare meat.

As to the infamous hasenpfeffer: it's a heavy, strongly flavored stew. In America, try making it with jackrabbit.

SLAUGHTER AND AFTER SLAUGHTER

Grocery stores rarely sell rabbit meat, but you can find it online or look up farmers markets, rabbit breeders, butchers, or specialty grocers. Buy locally if possible as the meat will be the freshest.

If you plan to raise and harvest your own rabbits, and have no experience with dressing animals, videos on the process are helpful but if at all possible, find a class or someone to show you in person. We have been learning through homesteaders' groups. We are very grateful to our homesteader friends Tom and Michelle who helped us the first time with our chickens and to Catherine B who walked us through processing our first rabbits. Videos are good. If that's what you have, I believe you can learn through them. But they *cannot* compare to having someone there to walk you through it.

I can't stress enough the importance of humane slaughter. The animal's stress releases hormones that can impact the taste and quality of the meat. Even if this were not so, of course, it is simply kind to limit a creature's pain in any way we possibly can.

Before you start, consider which parts of the animal you wish to keep. Many people don't want to eat the organs, but the liver, kidneys and heart *are* perfectly good to eat and are, by most people's judgment, delicious. If you don't want to eat them yourself, many people want them to make dog food.

If you want to keep the pelts, the skinning process is a little bit different.

Give your rabbits only water for about 24 to 36 hours before slaughter. They can be processed at any time, but it's better not to have food in their system. Be sure they are not pregnant.

While you can cook an animal immediately after slaughter, it's better to wait 24 hours after processing to put your rabbits in the freezer or eat them. Doing so earlier won't hurt you. The meat just may not be as tasty or tender.

JOINTING & SLAUGHTERING:

A cookbook cannot adequately cover the process of slaughtering and jointing a rabbit. If you plan on doing this yourself, please seek out a class, someone to teach you, or a multitude of videos freely available on the process. However, it's good to know the parts of the rabbit.

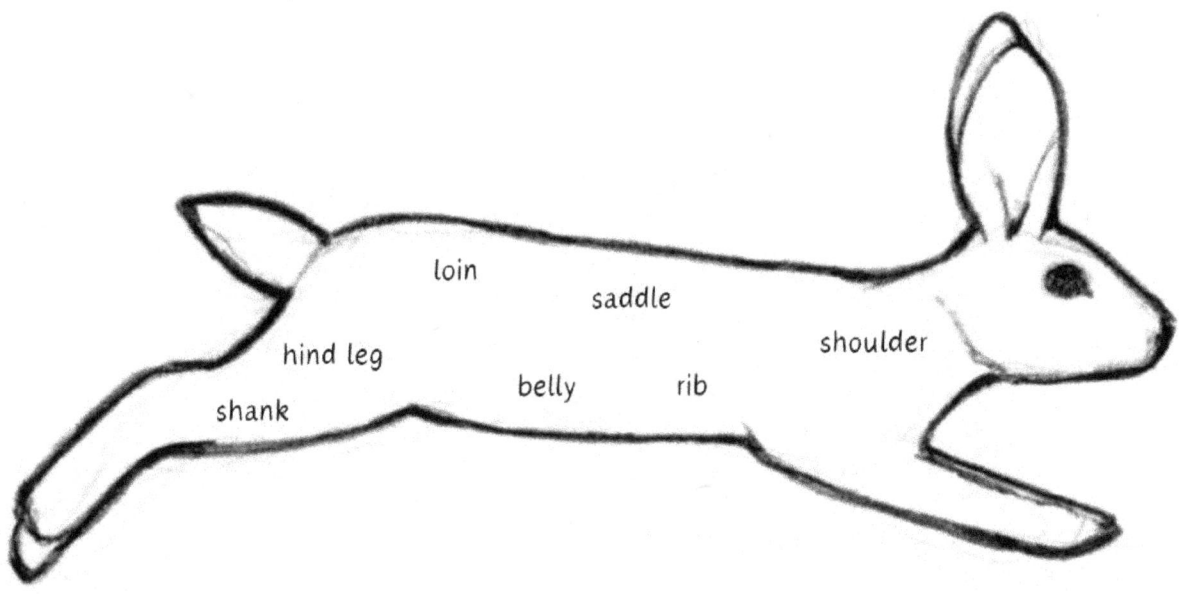

MODERN RECIPES

BRAISED

To braise food is to fry it lightly and then stew it slowly in a closed pot. Braising uses both wet and dry heat and distributes heat from all sides. The word comes from the French braise, *which means* live coals, *but the method is also often found in Asian cuisines.*

Porcini Braised Rabbit

Rabbit legs and liquid from this recipe are also used in the rabbit meatballs with Porcini tagliatelle recipe in the PASTA section.

INGREDIENTS	
1/4 ounce dried Porcinis, powdered	1/2 cup diced fennel bulb
1/4 ounce dried Porcinis	2 stalks celery, thickly sliced
1/2 cup white wine	2 carrots, thickly sliced
8 rabbit legs	1 onion, medium diced
6 cups rabbit or chicken stock	Salt & pepper

DIRECTIONS

1. Heat the oil in a pan. Rub the rabbit legs with porcini powder, salt, and pepper; then sear them in the hot oil. Flip as necessary until they're brown and crusty. Remove from pan and set aside.

2. Heat oil in a deep stock pot. Sauté the celery, carrot, onion, and fennel bulb until they're browned.

3. Deglaze the pot with white wine. Add the dried porcini and rabbit legs. Cover it with the rabbit or chicken stock. Place a circle or parchment paper with a slit cut in it over the pot.

4. Let the stock simmer, braising for an hour or until the legs are fork tender.

5. Strain the braising liquid and simmer it down on the stove until it's the consistency of a sauce.

6. Serve the sauce with the rabbit and any sides you like. Because it would be crazy to serve them with sides you *don't* like!

Braised Rabbit Pappardelle

PREP 30 minutes   COOK 1 hour 25 minutes   SERVES 5

INGREDIENTS

2 tablespoons olive oil	2 cups chicken stock
1 wild rabbit, jointed	18 ounces pappardelle pasta
4 slices smoked streaky bacon, chopped	Zest from 1/2 orange
1 small red onion, finely chopped	1 tablespoon Dijon mustard
1 carrot, finely chopped	1/3 cup double cream
3 garlic cloves, crushed	Small bunch flat-leaf parsley, chopped
2 rosemary sprigs, leaves picked and chopped	A few parsley leaves for garnish
1 tablespoon tomato purée	Grated Parmesan, to serve
2/3 cup white or rosé wine	

DIRECTIONS

1. Heat the oil in a large pan. When hot, add the rabbit, brown on all sides, then remove from the pan and set aside.

2. Add bacon, onion and carrot to the pan and cook for 10 mins until soft. Add garlic, rosemary and tomato purée, stir for 1-2 minutes, then pour in the wine and chicken stock.

3. Return the rabbit to the pan, season, cover with a lid and cook over low heat for an hour until the rabbit is really tender.

4. Remove the rabbit from the pan and shred the meat using 2 forks. Remove all the small bones. Increase the heat under the pan and boil anther 5 minutes until the liquid is reduced by half. Add the shredded meat and reduce the heat to low. Cook the pasta in a large pan of salted water. Drain, reserving a little pasta water to thin the sauce if necessary.

5. Stir half the orange zest, mustard, cream and parsley into the rabbit sauce. Add the cooked pasta to the pan, toss everything well to coat and heat through for 1-2 minutes. Serve in bowls with grated Parmesan, parsley leaves and the remaining orange zest.

Braised Rabbit with Tarragon, Mustard, and Cream

PREP 25 minutes   COOK 1 hour 30 minutes   SERVES 6

INGREDIENTS

4 pounds rabbit meat	2/3 cup dry white wine
1/4 cup plain flour	2/3 cup rabbit or chicken stock
2 tablespoons sunflower oil	1/2 rounded tablespoon wholegrain mustard
2 ounces unsalted butter	1/2 rounded tablespoon Dijon mustard
2 tablespoons tarragon vinegar/white wine vinegar	3 tablespoon double cream
4 garlic cloves, sliced	2 tablespoon chopped fresh tarragon
	Extra tarragon sprigs to garnish

DIRECTIONS

1. Season the rabbit pieces, then dust lightly with flour. Shake off the excess and save it. Heat the oil and half the butter in a large, deep frying pan over a medium heat until the butter is foaming. Add the rabbit pieces, a few at a time, and brown on both sides, then set aside on a plate. Pour away the excess fat; add vinegar and scrape the pan with a spatula to release all the caramelised bits. Pour this over the rabbit, then wipe the pan clean with paper towel.

2. Add the remaining butter to the pan. When it has melted, add the garlic and fry for 1 minute. Stir in the reserved flour, then gradually stir in the white wine and rabbit or chicken stock.

3. Return the rabbit pieces to the pan, cover tightly and simmer on low heat until tender: wild rabbit will take about 1-1¼ hours; farmed rabbit about 45 minutes.

4. Preheat the oven to 250 F

5. Lift the rabbit out onto a warmed serving dish with a slotted spoon, cover with foil and keep warm in the oven. Increase the heat under the pan on the stove and bubble for a few minutes until the liquid is slightly reduced and well flavored. Stir in the mustard and cream, then simmer a little longer until the sauce is just thick enough to lightly coat the back of a spoon. Taste, season and stir in the tarragon.

6. To serve, pour the sauce over the rabbit on the serving dish. Sprinkle with the extra tarragon sprigs, then serve with buttered mashed potato.

Cider Braised Rabbit

PREP 15 minutes   COOK 1 hour 15 minutes   SERVES 4

INGREDIENTS

1 rabbit, cut into 6-8 pieces	2 tablespoons butter
Flour to dust	2 cups cider
1 bulb fennel	8-1/2 cups chicken stock
2 leeks	2 cups small potatoes 300 g
1 carrot	1 tablespoon mustard
1 onion	Red wine vinegar, to taste
5 cloves garlic	1/3 bunch tarragon, finely chopped
5 bay leaves	1/3 bunch chervil, finely chopped
3 sprigs thyme	1/3 bunch parsley, finely chopped

DIRECTIONS

1. Flour the rabbit pieces and brown them in vegetable oil in a large pot over medium-high heat till lightly browned but not cooked, about 10 minutes.

2. Mince the vegetables and saute them in the same pan over medium heat until soft, about 5 minutes. Add butter, garlic, thyme, bay, cider, chicken stock and bring to a simmer.

3. Add the rabbit into the pot and cook for about an hour.

4. Cut potatoes into quarters and after 40 minutes,. Once cooked, take the rabbit pieces out and let the sauce thicken. Season with salt, pepper, mustard and vinegar. Add the rabbit back in and sprinkle with the chopped fresh herbs Voila! You are ready to serve! Most likely with cider.

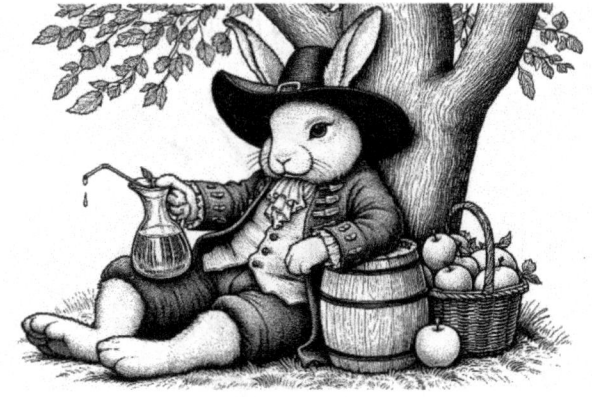

Rabbit Cacciotore (Italian, Braised)

'Cacciatore' means hunter in Italian.

PREP 30 minutes   COOK 1 hour 30 minutes   SERVES 4

INGREDIENTS

2 pounds of rabbit pieces	Large bunch parsley, chopped
2 tablespoons flour with salt and pepper	1-1/3 cups white wine
3 tablespoons olive oil	2 14 ounce cans cherry tomatoes
2 onions, chopped	20 large green olives
3 garlic cloves, chopped	1 tablespoon sugar

DIRECTIONS

1. Coat the rabbit in flour. Heat 1 tablespoon of olive oil in a large, shallow pan and brown the rabbit in 3 batches. Add oil for each batch. Set the rabbit aside.

2. Add onions and garlic to the pan with the remaining oil. Saute 15 minutes until softened. Add most of the parsley and cook for a few more minutes.

3. Return the rabbit to the pan and pour in the wine. Turn up the heat and simmer the wine until half-reduced, then stir in the cherry tomatoes. If the rabbit isn't completely covered, add a little water.

4. Cover the pan and simmer until the rabbit is tender, about 40 minutes, although the timing can vary. Add water as needed, cooking until the meat starts to come away from the bone.

5. When the meat is falling away from the bones, throw in the olives, cover and simmer for another 5-10 minutes. Season with sugar, salt and pepper, then sprinkle with the remaining parsley. Serve with polenta, mashed buttered potatoes or a buttery, flat pasta, such as tagliatelle

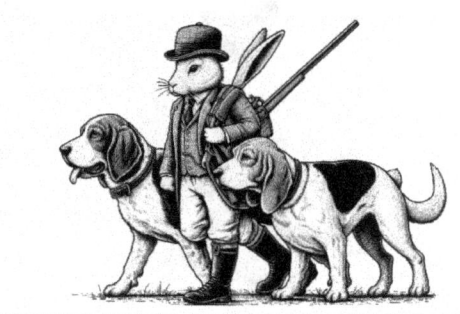

FRIED

Shawn's Fried Rabbit

PREP 45 minutes   COOK 30 minutes + 15 minutes frying   SERVES 2-3

INGREDIENTS

1 rabbit	2 cups flour
2 tablespoons salt	1/2 teaspoon salt
3 eggs, beaten	1/4 teaspoon pepper

DIRECTIONS

1. Cut the rabbit into pieces.
2. Fill a large pot about half way with water. Add 2 tablespoons of salt, and bring to a boil. Add rabbit, and parboil for 30 minutes. Drain, and let cool.
3. Beat eggs in a bowl. Not *into* the bowl. We want the eggs in the bowl, not you.
4. Mix flour with salt and pepper and put it in a shallow, wide plastic tub or bowl. Dip each rabbit piece first into the egg, and then the flour.
5. Heat 1/2" of oil in a large cast iron frying pan. When the oil is hot, turn the heat down to medium. Fry the rabbit pieces, one at a time in the oil. When first side is golden, flip it over. Cook until golden brown and crispy. Drain each piece on a paper towel, to soak up grease.
6. Serve hot with your favorite side dish. Preferably with potatoes or vegetables or something *on* the dish.

The American Rabbit Breeders Association recognizes more than 70 breeds of domestic rabbit and there are at least 305 domesticated breeds around the world. They range from the tiny Netherland Dwarf weighing in at 2 to 2-1/2 pounds up to the Flemish Giant and Continental Giants who can weigh in the low to mid-20 pound range!

Korean Extra Crispy Fried Rabbit

PREP 9-10 hours   COOK 20-25 minutes   SERVES 2-4

INGREDIENTS

1 pound rabbit	*Sauce*
1 cup buttermilk	1-1/2 tablespoons ketchup
1 teaspoon ground ginger	1 tablespoon gochujang (Korean fermented pepper paste)
1/2 teaspoon garlic powder	
1/2 teaspoon fine sea salt	2 tablespoons honey
1/2 cup corn starch, plus extra	1 tablespoon sugar
Peanut oil for frying	1 tablespoon soy sauce
Toasted sesame seeds for garnish	1 teaspoon toasted sesame seed oil
Chopped green onion for garnish	

DIRECTIONS

1. Remove as much silver skin as possible. Cut the rabbit into 6-8 sections. You can debone the loins but they hold moisture better when cooked on the bone. Place rabbit pieces in a large bowl, completely covered with buttermilk. Cover the bowl and set in the refrigerator overnight.

2. Strain rabbit from buttermilk and season with ginger, garlic powder, and 1/2 teaspoon of fine sea salt. In a small bowl, mix sauce ingredients together until smooth and set aside. If you want dipping sauce, double the recipe.

3. Pour 2 inches of peanut oil into a pot and heat to 350°F.

4. Coat rabbit in corn starch, shaking off excess. Fry rabbit 3 to 5 minutes, until the coating starts to harden and is light brown. Remove from oil and set aside. Return the oil to 350°F before each batch. Don't crowd the pan, and don't let the oil get lower than 300°F when frying.

5. After all the rabbit has been fried once, return oil to 350°F and fry each piece again, until they turn golden and have an internal temperature of at least 155°F. Drain on a rack.

6. Toss the fried rabbit with the sauce in a large bowl. Garnish with sesame seed and green onion and serve!

Buttermilk Fried Rabbit

If using wild cottontails, brine before frying in 1/4 cup kosher salt to 4 cups water. Submerge your rabbit in brine for 8 hours to keep them moist. Domesticated rabbits don't need this, but if you want to brine them, do so for no more than 4 hours.

PREP 4-9 hours   COOK 25 minutes   SERVES: 4

INGREDIENTS

2 to 4 rabbits, cut into serving pieces	2 teaspoons cayenne, or to taste
2 cups buttermilk	1 1/2 cups flour
2 tablespoons Italian seasoning *	1 teaspoon salt
1 tablespoon paprika	2 cups vegetable oil
1 tablespoon garlic powder	

* or mix together 1 1/2 teaspoons oregano, 1 1/2 teaspoons thyme and 1 tablespoon dried parsley

DIRECTIONS

1. Mix the buttermilk and all the spices except the salt and flour. Coat the rabbit with the buttermilk mix and set in a covered container for at least four hours. Overnight is better.
2. Pour the oil into a large cast iron pan, about an inch deep. The oil should go halfway up the side of the rabbit. Turn the heat to medium-high.

Frying – frying needs to be done in batches. Flour pieces immediately before frying.
1. Remove the rabbit from the buttermilk and leave it in a strainer to drain.
2. Heat the oil until a sprinkle of flour immediately sizzles, about 325°F.
3. Shake flour and salt together in a plastic bag. Add a few pieces of rabbit and shake to coat.
4. Put the coated pieces in a single layer in the hot oil. They shouldn't touch one another. Fry 8 to 12 minutes keeping the oil at a steady sizzle. Turn over and fry for about another 10 minutes, until they're golden brown. The forelegs will be done first, then the loin, and lastly the hind legs.
5. When the pieces are fried, set them on a rack over a paper towel to drain excess oil. Keep the early batches in a warm oven.

Mom's Fried Rabbit & Gravy

INGREDIENTS

1 rabbit, cut into serving pieces	3 tablespoons all-purpose flour
1/3 cup all-purpose flour	1-1/2 cups milk or chicken broth
1/2 teaspoon salt	Salt and pepper
1/8 teaspoon black pepper	Worcestershire sauce (or Kitchen bouquet, Gravy
Vegetable oil for frying	Master, Parisian Essence or any browning sauce)

DIRECTIONS

1. In a shallow pan, combine 1/3 cup of flour, salt, pepper, and cayenne pepper and mix well. Add rabbit pieces, coating well.

2. In a large skillet, heat 1/4 inch of oil over medium-high heat. When it's hot, add coated meat and brown it on all sides.

3. Reduce heat and cover. Cook over very low heat for 20-25 minutes, turning once, until tender.

4. Remove cover. Cook 5 minutes longer to crisp the meat.

5. Set meat aside on a paper-towel lined plate and cover to keep warm.

6. Save 3 tablespoons of the oil, on medium heat. Stir 3 tablespoons of flour into the oil. Stir in milk or broth. Cook over medium heat, stirring constantly, until it thickens and bubbles. Add salt, pepper, and browning sauce to taste.

GRILLED

Some basic tips on grilling rabbit:

Fresh is best. Remove excess fat and silver skin. Use a sharp knife. Rinse the rabbit well under cold running water and pat dry with paper towels. Marinate in the refrigerator for at least 2 hours. Overnight is better.

Good marinades for rabbits might use olive oil, lemon juice, rosemary, garlic and salt. Marinades enhance the flavor and also help break down muscle fiber. Lemon tenderizes the meat and leaves it quite succulent. Avoid heavy spices. Rabbit has a delicate flavor that can be easily overpowered.

A simple marinade is salt, pepper, and minced garlic. Or try a blend of fresh herbs. Try rosemary, thyme, sage, and oregano mixed with olive oil, garlic, salt, and pepper.

For some spice, use chili peppers mixed with olive oil, garlic, salt, and pepper or just sprinkle cayenne pepper directly on the meat.

For an Asian flavor, try soy sauce and ginger mixed in honey.

Other options can include mustards, citrus flavors or beer or wine bases.

When the grill is hot, about 325 to 350 F, remove the rabbit from the marinade. Grill 6-8 minutes per side, or 12-15 minutes/pound. Look for an internal temperature of 160 ° F. A medium high heat helps lock in moisture and keep the meat tender.

If possible, use indirect heat, placing rabbit on the grill farthest from the heat source.

Flip the rabbit frequently to prevent burning and for even cooking. Basting with marinade or olive oil while grilling helps the meat to stay moist.

Let the rabbi rest for a few minutes after grilling.

Mustard and Bacon Grilled Rabbit

PREP 2 hours, 15 minutes   COOK 1 hour   SERVES 4

INGREDIENTS

1 shallot diced	Freshly ground black pepper
2 garlic cloves garlic, minced	3 pounds whole rabbit
2 tablespoons olive oil	10 to 12 bacon slices
4 tablespoons Dijon mustard	Herbs for garnish
Pinch of sea salt	

DIRECTIONS

1. Blend shallot, garlic, olive oil, and mustard in a bowl. Put the rabbit in a non-reactive baking dish and rub it all over with the sauce. Cover and let sit at room temperature for at least 2 hours or refrigerate it, covered, overnight. Remove from the refrigerator at least 2 hours before grilling.

2. Build a medium size fire in the barbecue or light the gas grill using the 2 outside burners. When the coals are red and dusted with ash, divide them in the barbecue, putting half the coals on either side. Put a grill pan in the center of the barbecue to catch any drippings.

3. Season the marinated rabbit with salt and pepper, wrap it with the bacon strips and tie or skewer them into place.

4. Put the grill over the coals. When it is hot, place the rabbit directly on the grill over the drip pan. Turn it every 15 minutes, or as often as necessary to prevent burning on any side, until it is cooked through which should take an hour. Half way through cooking, brush the rabbit with any remaining mustard sauce.

5. When the rabbit is cooked, let it rest on a cutting board for 10 minutes before removing the string, and cutting the rabbit into serving pieces. Cut the bacon into large bite-sized pieces.

6. If you have the liver, rub it all over with oil and place it on the grill until it is golden on all sides and slightly rosy inside, 6 to 7 minutes. Remove from the grill and season with salt and pepper and cut into pieces.

7. Set the rabbit pieces and bacon on a platter. Arrange liver pieces on the platter, garnish with bay leaves or other herbs, and serve.

Grilled and Marinated Garlic Rabbit

PREP 40 minutes   COOK 40 minutes   SERVES 2

INGREDIENTS

2-1/2 pounds rabbit, cut up (wild rabbits are best)	1 teaspoon honey
Fresh thyme and rosemary sprigs	4 thick slices of pancetta or bacon
4 garlic cloves, peeled	Sea salt
Olive oil	Freshly ground black pepper
Grated zest and juice of 1 untreated lemon	5 skewers

DIRECTIONS

1. Soak the skewers in water. Preheat the oven to 400 F or use the grill.

2. Put the meat in a bowl.

3. Remove the leaves off the thyme and rosemary sprigs. Mix them into a paste in a mortar or blender. Add the garlic and chop finely. Stir in 8 tablespoons of olive oil, lemon zest and juice, and honey. Pour the marinade over the meat and set aside for 25 minutes.

4. Remove the meat from the marinade. Season with salt and pepper. Put 2 slices of bacon between the belly flaps and fix the "sandwich" with 3 skewers. Place the legs and barrels on the grill. After 10 minutes, add the prepared belly piece, after another 10 minutes the back and rib pieces. Turn all the pieces regularly, using fresh sprigs to brush them with the marinade each time. Keep an eye on the grill heat. If you're using the oven, bake them for the same amounts of time.

5. Cut the kidneys three quarters deep and open them like a book. Cut the liver into 4 pieces. Put each kidney between 2 pieces of liver and secure with a skewer.

6. When the pieces on the grill are done, move them to the edge of the grill grate where it's not as hot. Lay the skewers with the innards and the last 2 bacon slices on the grill. When it's crispy, in a few minutes, place the bacon over the pieces of meat.

7. Serve with white beans or fried potatoes, salads or grilled vegetables, and white wine. Do not forget the white wine!

BBQ Grilled Rabbit with Mashed Potatoes

PREP 5-25 hours   COOK 30 minutes   SERVES 4-6

INGREDIENTS

Rabbit Marinade	*Mashed Potatoes*
5 cloves of garlic	5 large potatoes
1/2 white onion	1 whole stick of butter
1/4 Cup parsley	1 whole cream cheese
1/2 lime juice	Milk to taste (Until creamy)
3 tablespoons olive oil	Salt to taste
2 teaspoons smoked paprika	
Black pepper and salt to taste	
2-3 pounds rabbit meat	

DIRECTIONS

1. *Rabbit Marinade:* Grind garlic, parsley, lime juice, cilantro, olive oil, and salt and pepper together in a mortar. Add onions and paprika and grind well. Slash meat to allow marinade to penetrate meat. Brush marinade on and let sit for 5 to 24 hours.

2. *Potatoes:* Peel, chop, and boil potatoes in salted water seasoned. When tender, drain water, put potatoes back in the hot pot and mash with butter, cream cheese, and milk.

3. *Basting Rabbit Sauce*: Mix together 1/2 stick of salted butter, 1 teaspoon smoked paprika, 3 crushed garlics mixed with 1 tbs sugar

4. Set grill to 350 F and grill until you have an internal temperature of 160 F. Baste with rabbit sauce while grilling. Cover grill and baste again. Repeat as desired.

5. Serve cooked rabbit on a bed of mashed potatoes, sprinkled with green onion tops, sliced thin.

PORCHETTA

Porchetta is typically a rolled meat dish made from pork and seasoned with garlic, fennel, and herbs, rolled, tied, and roasted. The same form can be used with rabbit. It is of a size, however, better suited for a family dinner and can be prepared in much less time.

Rabbit Porchetta

PREP 1-3 days   COOK 45 minutes   SERVES

INGREDIENTS

1 large stewed rabbit, 4 to 6 pounds	Sea salt
2 tablespoons extra virgin olive oil	4 cloves of garlic
Freshly ground black pepper	Zest of 2 lemons
1 tablespoon fennel pollen	1/2 cup chopped herbs*

* one suggestion would be rosemary, oregano, parsley, sage

DIRECTIONS:

1. Preheat oven to 425 F.

2. Pound the garlic to a fine paste in a mortar and pestle.

3. Bone the rabbit. Remove kidneys and liver with a sharp knife and set aside. Remove the forelegs from the body. Save them for another use. Starting at the neck, remove the meat from the bone. When you reach the loin area, curve the tip of your knife around the loin until you hit the backbone. Repeat this process down the length of the rib cage until you reach the back legs. Remove the backbone by severing the tip of each vertebra while simultaneously pulling the rib cage away from the rabbit. Take care not to pierce through the meat. Separate the leg bones from the hip socket by carefully popping them out of the socket from behind. Remove the bones from the legs on both sides, taking care to only cut as deep as the bone.

4. Lay the boneless rabbit out flat and rub the inside with the pounded garlic and lemon zest. Season inside and out with salt, pepper and fennel pollen. Sprinkle herbs over the interior. Roll the boneless rabbit tightly around itself lengthwise. Tie with butcher's twine at 3-inch intervals. Wrap tightly with plastic wrap and refrigerate for one to three days.

5. Set the rabbit on a rack in a roasting pan. Rub a light layer of olive oil all over. Roast for 45 minutes or until a meat thermometer says 140°F in the thickest portion of the roast. After removing from the oven, allow the roast to sit for 10 minutes before slicing it into half-inch rounds. Strain the pan juices and spoon them over the sliced meat.

Porchetta #2

This is a *very* ambitious meal! There are four parts to it, *lots* of prep, lots of chilling time. I included it, first, because I felt each type of recipe should show a variety of ways to make it. Second, it's fun to have a challenging option! Third and most important is that there are almost no rabbit porchettas anywhere on the internet. You can, of course, substitute rabbit for any pork porchetta, of which you *can* find thousands. But knowing something about the types of foods (in this case meats) you're substituting for can impact your choices in seasoning, cooking methods, etc. See the third porchetta recipe for a comparison of rabbit meat and pork meat.

PREP 12-24 hours   COOK 1-1/2 hours   SERVES 3-4

INGREDIENTS

Rabbit

1 whole rabbit, with its livers

1 lemon, zested

1 teaspoon ground caraway

1 teaspoon fennel pollen

4 garlic cloves, ground to a paste with extra virgin olive oil

1/4 cup chopped curly parsley

Salt and pepper, to taste

As needed - Activa RM (transglutaminase or "meat glue")

Rabbit Liver Mousse

2 large rabbit livers

Cold butter, diced, equal to the weight of the livers)

1 garlic clove, peeled and sliced

1 shallot, peeled and sliced

1 pinch chili flakes

1 tablespoon. Dijon mustard

Salt, to taste

1/4 cup aquavit

Oil-butter blend, for sautéing

Rabbit Jus

2 yellow onions, chopped

2 celery ribs, chopped

2 carrots, chopped

1 bunch fresh thyme

1 tablespoon black peppercorns

1 bulb garlic, coarsely chopped

3-4 bay leaves

1 quart chicken stock

1 3/4 gallon water

1/4 cup Dijon mustard

Lemon juice to taste

1 cup crème fraiche

Salt, pepper, to taste

Vegetables

1 1/4 lbs. assorted rainbow carrots, peeled, halved and cooked

1 pound. fingerling potatoes, peeled and cooked

1 heaping tsp. ground caraway seed

1/4 pound butter

1 large handful curly parsley, coarsely chopped

DIRECTIONS

Rabbit

1. Remove back legs, debone and pound flat.

2. Have two rabbit halves, each with loin, tenderloin, and front leg. For each half, remove loin and tenderloin from belly.

3. Season all four legs and the belly meat with all the seasons and herbs in the rabbit ingredients, except Activa.

4. Cook the front legs sous vide with water at 180 F with 1 tablespoon of butter, for six hours, then chill.

5. Dust back legs with Activa and wrap the leg meat around the loin and tenderloin. Place the leg roll on the edge of the belly meat, dust with Activa and roll the legs in the belly meat. Repeat with the other leg and belly. Wrap each porchetta in plastic wrap; twist to tighten. Refrigerate overnight.

Rabbit Liver Mousse

1. Heat butter and oil in a saute pan until very hot. Add livers. Sear on both sides. Do not overcook. They should be no more than medium. Remove the livers, drain the oil and put the pan back on the heat.

2. Add the extra butter, garlic, shallot, and chili flakes. Turn the heat down and saute vegetables until they're soft.

3. Add aquavit; reduce until almost dry.

4. Place the reduction, while still hot, into a blender with livers and Dijon mustard and puree until smooth. Leaving the blender running, add cold butter a cube at a time to emulsify. Pour the mousse into a container and set it in the refrigerator to chill.

Rabbit Jus

1. Roast the rabbit bones with vegetables, aromatics, chicken stock and water to make a stock. Simmer 3 to 4 hours.

2. Strain the stock and reduce it to 2 cups of thick, dark rabbit stock.

3. Whisk in 1/4 cup Dijon mustard and 1 cup *dreme fraiche*. Season as desired with salt, pepper, and fresh lemon juice.

Putting it All Together

1. In a sauté pan large enough for the vegetables, both porchettas, and both front legs, heat a small amount of oil in it until very hot.

2. Brown the porchetta in the heated oil and brown evenly all around. Remove and set it aside.

3. Add the front legs and brown the side that will be presented. Remove and drain oil from the pan.

4. Add 1/4 pound of butter and melt it. Put in the carrots, potatoes, and caraway. Salt the vegetables and toss them to coat them in hot butter.

5. Add all the rabbit back into the pan. Set it in an oven preheated to 425 F for about 15 minute until it's hot and golden brown.

6. Remove the rabbit from the pan and set it aside.

7. Toss the vegetables with curly parsley and season it with lemon juice. Put them on a warm platter and pour half the rabbit jus on either side of the vegetables.

8. Slice the porchettas, and set one on each side of the vegetables. Place one leg on either side of the vegetables. Garnish it with the rabbit liver spread on baguette and carrot greens.

9. Serve with a carafe of the remaining rabbit jus.

In many cultures and faiths from Christianity to ancient Egypt to American Indians and the Aztecs and Mayans, rabbits have been seen as a symbol of fertility, abundance, renewal, and rebirth.

Substituting Rabbit for Pork

This recipe originally called for pork but can be made with rabbit. It would be fun to try making it both ways to compare.

The difference between rabbit and pork is that rabbit is healthier and leaner, with fewer calories per ounce and more protein. It has a more delicate flavor—although the flavor will be impacted both by the rabbit's diet and by its age. An older rabbit will be gamier and the meat may be tougher and require longer stewing and more tenderizing.

The differences mean you must be more careful not to let the rabbit meat become tough or dry while cooking. Some suggestions:

Roast rabbit meat at 350 F for 20-25 minutes per pound. Baste it with butter or oil for moistness. This is a little higher than pork, for which 325 F is recommended.

Braise rabbit by cooking in broth, wine, or any liquid, for an hour or two to keep the meat tender.

For **grilling**, it's best to marinate rabbit first for flavor and moisture, then use medium-high heat for 5-7 minutes per side. Marinating is also recommended for pork, but suggested grilling time is slightly less at 4-6 minutes per side.

Italian Pork Porchetta

This recipe is for an Italian pork porchetta with rabbit substituted.

INGREDIENTS

4 pounds boneless rabbit belly, skin on	4 cloves fresh garlic minced
1 pound rabbit tenderloin	1 tablespoon fennel pollen
2 tablespoons dried sage, chopped	2 tablespoons Kosher salt
2 tablespoons fresh rosemary, chopped	1 tablespoon black peppercorns
2 tablespoons extra virgin olive oil	

DIRECTIONS

1. Preheat the oven to 350 F.
2. Lay the rabbit skin side down on a cutting board. With a sharp knife make a few slits in the flesh. Make a lengthwise slit on the tenderloin.
3. Mix together sage, rosemary garlic, salt, and olive oil. Spread the marinade over the surface of the belly, making sure it gets into the cuts in the flesh.
4. Sprinkle fennel pollen over the belly and tenderloin.
5. Lay the tenderloin in the middle of the pork belly. Roll the belly around the tenderloin and tie with butcher's twin. Put it in a roasting pan.
6. Make slits in the skin with a sharp knife. Drizzle more olive oil over the porchetta and sprinkle with salt and pepper.
7. Cook in the oven for 2-1/2 to 3 hours. It's done when poking with a knife results in juices running clear.

ROASTED & BAKED

There are differences between roasting and baking. Roasting is typically done at a higher temperature than baking—400 F or higher. Baking is usually only up to 375 F and is more likely to call for covering the food. Some say that roasting involves a food or foods that are already what they are and will not meld or join, as opposed to a casserole or bread or cookies where the different ingredients bake together into something new.

However, the words are often used interchangeably. So I'll include the roasted and baked rabbit in one section, labeling each recipe as it was labeled where I found it.

Roasted Rabbit in Wine Sauce and Garlic

PREP 15 minutes   COOK 15 minutes   SERVES 3-4

INGREDIENTS

1 tablespoon olive oil or sunflower oil	1/2 cup chicken stock
1-1/2 pounds rabbit's 3 cloves of garlic	Sea salt
1 cup of dry white wine	Fresh thyme
Splash of water	1 rabbit

DIRECTIONS

1. Preheat oven to 350 F.
2. Chop the garlic. Cut the rabbit into four legs and two pieces for the body.
3. Heat a large pan on medium-high heat and add oil. Add the rabbit pieces and sear them on all sides until well browned (5 minutes per side). Don't turn too often. Season with salt and pepper while it's cooking.
4. Reduce the heat slightly. Add chopped garlic and brown it while continuing to cook rabbit, about 2-3 minutes. Turn the heat to medium. Season the rabbit again and deglaze with white wine to get all the caramelized juices from the bottom of the pan. After the wine evaporates, you'll have a syrupy substance left. Add chicken stock.
5. Put the pan with the rabbit pieces into the preheated oven and roast for about 30 minutes until the internal temperature is 140 to 145°F. Serve with fresh thyme as a garnish.

*The wine garlic sauce should be reduced quite a bit to intensify the flavor. It should end up not too thick, but not too runny. When cooking, add a little bit of water when cooking. Do not add chicken stock or the stock flavor will be too strong.

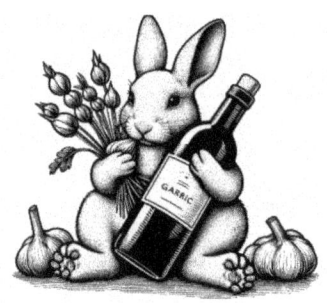

Roasted Rabbit with Olive and Feta

PREP 45 minutes, plus 1 hour marinating   COOK   SERVES 2 to 4

INGREDIENTS

1 3-pound rabbit, cut into 8 pieces	1/2 cup white wine, not too dry, such as Riesling
1 tablespoon chopped fresh rosemary	1 tablespoon extra-virgin olive oil
2 teaspoons chopped fresh oregano	5 thin slices lemon, seeded
6 garlic cloves, crushed and peeled	1/4 cup pitted kalamata olives, halved
2 teaspoons kosher salt, more to taste	4 tablespoons unsalted butter, cut into pieces
1/2 teaspoon black pepper	4 ounces feta cheese, preferably French, crumbled

DIRECTIONS

1. Preheat oven to 400 F.

2. Put rabbit pieces in a large bowl; toss with rosemary, oregano, garlic, salt and pepper. Cover loosely with plastic wrap and let stand at room temperature for 1 hour.

3. Simmer wine in a small saucepan over medium heat until it's reduced by half.

4. Heat oil in a large skillet over medium-high heat. Add rabbit and garlic in a single layer and cook until meat is golden brown, 3 to 4 minutes a side. If the garlic gets too dark before the rabbit is finished browning, put the garlic on top of the rabbit to keep it from cooking more.

5. Put lemon slices, olives and half the butter into the pan. Pour in reduced wine. Cover and put it in the oven for 5 minutes. Uncover and scatter feta over top. Return to oven until rabbit is just cooked through, 5 to 10 minutes more. Stir in remaining butter, salt to taste and serve.

Baked Rabbit & Chorizo Rice

PREP marinating time + 20 minutes COOK 1 hour   SERVES 6

INGREDIENTS

1 rabbit, portioned	1/2 teaspoon smoked paprika
4 ounces (a glass) of white wine	1 tablespoon tomato purée
1 tablespoon olive oil, plus extra for frying	7 ounces paella rice
A bunch of thyme	3-1/2 cups fresh chicken stock
1-1/3 cups chorizo	Pinch of saffron
1 onion, chopped	7 ounces frozen peas
3 garlic cloves, sliced	Parsley, chopped

DIRECTIONS

1. Preheat oven to 350 F.

2. Soak the saffron in 2 tablespoons of boiling water.

3. Cut the rabbit into about 20 small pieces. Or 19. Or 21. Marinate the meat in the wine, olive oil and thyme for a minimum of one hour. Overnight is better.

4. Drain the rabbit from the marinade, reserving the liquid. Heat some oil in a shallow casserole dish and sizzle the chorizo until crisp. Remove the chorizo and drain the excess oil.

5. Brown the rabbit pieces in 2 batches and set aside. Add the onion and garlic, cook until soft, then stir in the paprika and tomato purée. Stir in the rice, then pour the reserved marinade, the stock and saffron over it.

6. Nestle the rabbit into the rice with the chorizo, cover, bring to the boil, then bake for 40-50 minutes, until the rice and rabbit are tender and all the liquid has been absorbed. Stir in the frozen peas to defrost.

7. Garnish with parsley and serve!

Baked Rabbit with Apple and Lemon

PREP 10 minutes   COOK 60 minutes   SERVES 4

INGREDIENTS

2-1/4 pounds rabbit cut into pieces	6 cloves of garlic
2 apples	1/2 cup olive oil
1 lemon	1/2 cup butter, cut into pieces
Juice of one lemon	2 bay leaves
Pepper to taste	Salt to taste
Nutmeg to taste	

DIRECTIONS

1. Preheat oven to 350 F.
2. Wash and quarter the apples and lemons.
3. Put rabbit pieces in a baking dish. Season with salt, lemon juice, pepper, nutmeg, bay leaf, peeled garlic and the quartered apples and lemon. Add margarine pieces and drizzle olive oil over it all.
4. Bake for one hour, occasionally basting the rabbit with the sauce.

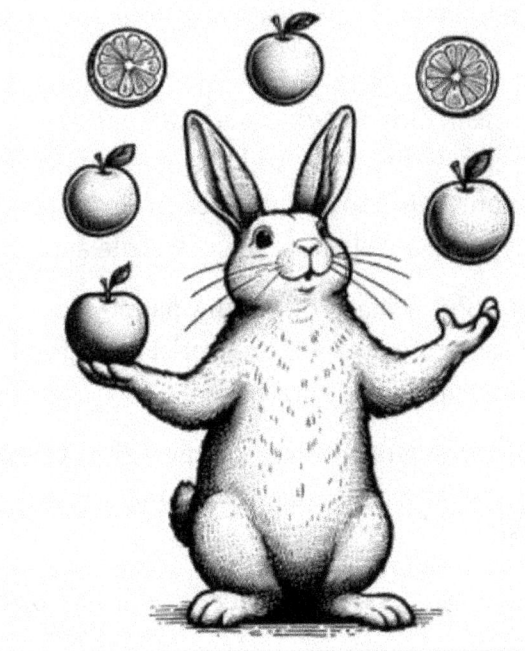

Baked Rabbit in Mustard Sauce

PREP 20minutes   COOK 2 hours   SERVES 6

INGREDIENTS

1 large rabbit jointed into 6 portions	1 teaspoon Dijon Mustard
2 large shallots finely sliced	2 cups Chicken stock
2 teaspoons plain flour	1/3 cup double cream
2 ounces Butter	2 sprigs fresh thyme
1 teaspoons olive oil	1 bay leaf
3/4 to 1 cup of white wine	

DIRECTIONS

1. Preheat the oven to 350°F.

2. Melt half the butter with the oil in a large frying pan over medium heat. Season the rabbit with salt and black pepper; then sauté them to golden brown on all sides. Move the rabbit to a large casserole dish.

3. Wipe the frying pan clean. Add the remaining butter, turn the heat to medium and sauté the sliced shallots until softened, about 5 minutes. Add flour to the shallots, stirring continuously, for 1 minute.

4. Remove the pan from the heat. Stir in wine and half the stock. Return the pan to the heat, stirring constantly until the sauce thickens. Add the mustard, season with salt and black pepper and simmer on low for 2 minutes. Remove the sauce from the heat and pour it over the rabbit in the casserole dish. Add the remaining stock to the casserole and bring it to a boil on the stove.

5. Add the thyme and bay leaf. Put a piece of baking parchment on the surface of the casserole, and put the lid on. Put the casserole into the preheated oven for 1.5 hours, or until tender – the meat will begin to fall off the bone when cooked.

6. Remove the casserole from the oven and place on the stove. Use a slotted spoon to remove the rabbit pieces and set them aside. Stir in the cream and simmer for 5 minutes, removing the sprigs of thyme and bay leaf.

7. Replace the rabbit pieces and season to taste. Serve on a bed of cabbage with potatoes of any sort and green vegetables.

STEWS

Rabbit and Dumplings

PREP 1 hour   COOK 1 hour 30 minutes   SERVES 8+

INGREDIENTS

For the rabbit:

2 whole rabbits

1/2 gallon mirepoix (onion, carrot, celery)

2 cups white wine

3/4 gallon chicken stock

2 cups large diced carrots

2 cups large diced celery root

2 cups large diced celery

2 cups large diced turnips

2 cups large diced onion

3/4 stick butter, divided

2 tablespoons freshly chopped rosemary leaves

2 tablespoons freshly chopped thyme leaves

2 tablespoons freshly chopped sage leaves

2 tablespoons freshly chopped garlic

1/2 cup all-purpose flour

Salt and freshly ground black pepper

Hot sauce

Worcestershire sauce

Dried thyme

Dumplings:

1 cup all-purpose flour

Salt and freshly ground black pepper

Pinch ground cayenne

Pinch ground nutmeg

Pinch rubbed sage

1 tablespoon baking powder

1 tablespoon melted butter

2 eggs

1/2 cup buttermilk

DIRECTIONS

1. Sear the rabbits in a large skillet over medium-high heat. Add mirepoix and caramelize.
2. Deglaze the pan with the wine. Add stock and simmer until rabbit is tender.
3. Let the rabbit cool, then pick the meat off the bones. Reserve the juice.
4. Sear vegetables in about 1/4 stick butter, until lightly browned. Add herbs, garlic and wine. Reduce until the pan is almost dry.
5. Add 1/2 stick butter; stir to melt without breaking. Stir in the flour until incorporated. Gradually stir in reserved juice.

6. Cook about 30 minutes until roux taste is gone. Add rabbit meat and season, to taste, with salt, pepper, hot sauce, Worcestershire sauce and dried thyme.

7. Preheat the oven to 375 degrees F.

8. Mix all dry ingredients. Mix all wet ingredients. Mix dry and wet ingredients together, stirring as little as possible.

9. Pour the stew in a large casserole dish and drop golf ball size dumplings all over the top.

10. Bake in preheated oven for 20 to 30 minutes, until bubbling around the edges and the dumplings have become golden brown on top.

Brer Rabbit was the star of many stories told by Uncle Remus to the children gathered at his feet, in the books written by Joel Chandler Harris in the late 1800s. Although Harris became accomplished in later life as an editor, folklorist, and author, he was very conscious of his status as an illegitimate child. When he started working for the newspaper on a plantation at the age of 14, he spent a great deal of time in the slaves' quarters where he felt more accepted and there, learned many of their stories passed down orally. These, he preserved and told in the books he would later write.

Brer Rabbit is a wily character, a bit of a trickster, who shows that one does not necessarily need strength or brawn to win, as he uses his wits in story after story to outsmart Brer Fox and Brer Wolf. The stories were known in several African countries although the Akan features the same stories with Anansi the spider as the trickster. Anansi does, in several stories, meet a trickster rabbit named Adanko.

German Rabbit Stew

This is a Swabian recipe, from Southern Germany, although the lemon, capers, and bay leaves give it a Greek feel. The Germans, however, replace the oregano, olive oil, and yogurt, with parsley, butter and sour cream. It is brothy, meaty and tart, with just a touch of creaminess.

This is a two-step stew. You first make the base, then add sour cream, white wine and capers right at the end. If you want to prepare this for multiple meals ahead of time, stop at step 4 to store just the base and add the remaining ingredients when you want to eat.

INGREDIENTS

2 cottontail rabbits or 1 domestic rabbit	2 to 3 bay leaves
Salt	1/4 cup lemon juice
2 tablespoons unsalted butter	2 tablespoons capers
2 tablespoons flour	1/2 cup sour cream
1 to 2 cups chicken stock	2 tablespoons white wine or to taste
1 onion, sliced root to tip	Black pepper
Lemon zest, white pith removed, cut into wide strips	Parsley to garnish

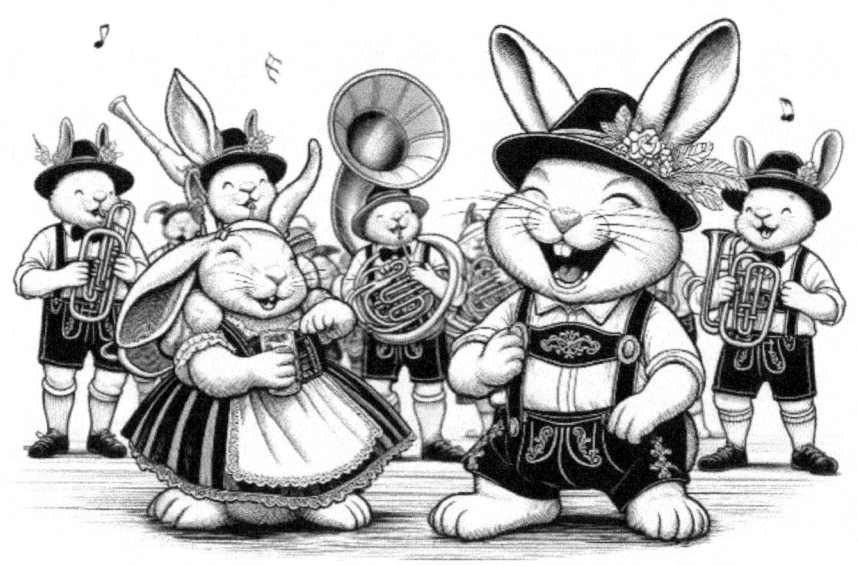

DIRECTIONS

1. Cut rabbits into pieces. Salt them well and set aside for about 10 minutes. Set a heavy, lidded pot over medium-high heat. Add a tablespoon of butter. Pat the rabbit pieces dry and brown them well on all sides. You may need to do this in batches. Don't crowd the pot. Remove the rabbit pieces once they're browned. This may take 15 minutes or so.

2. Add the remaining tablespoon of butter, then the sliced onion and cook until the edges just begin to brown, about 6 minutes. Sprinkle with flour and stir well. Cook, stirring often, until the flour turns golden, about 5 minutes.

3. Return the rabbit to the pot and add enough chicken stock to cover. Use a wooden spoon to scrape any browned bits off the bottom of the pot. Add the lemon zest, bay leaves and lemon juice and bring to a simmer. Cover and cook on low until the rabbit begins to fall off the bone—90 minutes to 3 hours, depending on how old your rabbit was. If you decided to cook a 10-year-old rabbit, settle in with some snacks to tide you over for a couple days or more.

4. Turn off the heat, remove the rabbit pieces and let them cool on a baking sheet. Pull all the meat off the bones and return the meat to the stew. (Or optionally, leave it all on the bone.)

5. You can save the stew or serve it immediately. Turn the heat to low to make sure the stew is nice and hot. Do not let it simmer. Add the sour cream, capers and as much white wine as you want. Stir in plenty of black pepper and garnish with parsley.

6. Serve with bread or potatoes and a crisp German white wine or lager beer.

Slow-Cooked Rabbit Stew

This slow-cooked rabbit stew has rich flavors from prunes, brandy and herbs.

PREP 25 minutes   COOK 2 hours 10 minutes   SERVES 4

INGREDIENTS

5 ounces prunes	1 onion, chopped
2 ounces brandy	2 celery sticks, chopped
2 ounces soft brown sugar	1 garlic clove, crushed
2 rabbits, jointed	2 thyme sprigs
Plain flour, for dusting	1 bay leaf
1 tablespoons vegetable oil	2/3 cup good red wine
3 slices of smoked bacon in thin strips	1 cup chicken stock
2 carrots, chopped	Chopped parsley and wild rice, to serve

DIRECTIONS

1. Heat oven to 300 F.
2. Put the prunes in a bowl with the brandy and brown sugar, stir, then set aside to soak.
3. Coat the rabbit in the flour. Heat the oil in a large pan and brown the rabbit all over until golden. Set the rabbit aside. Add the bacon, vegetables, garlic and herbs to the dish and fry for 5 minutes until starting to brown and soften.
4. Pour in the red wine and scrape everything off the bottom of the dish. Add the chicken stock and put the rabbit back in the dish with the prunes. Cover and cook for 2 hours, stirring occasionally, until the rabbit is totally tender.
5. Serve scattered with parsley and wild rice on the side.

Ischian Rabbit Stew, Italian

This is a traditional rabbit stew from the Italian island of Ischia, topped with a gremolata, typically made from lemon, parsley and finely chopped garlic.

INGREDIENTS

Extra-virgin olive oil	2 bay leaves
1 rabbit, about 3 pounds, jointed	A few sprigs thyme
1 onion, finely diced	7 ounces cherry tomatoes
2 cloves garlic, sliced	Gremolata
1 teaspoon chili flakes	A small bunch flat-leaf parsley, finely chopped
2 tablespoons tomato purée	1 clove garlic, finely chopped
2 cups white wine	1 lemon, zested and 1/2 juiced
1-1/2 cups chicken stock	1/2 cup extra-virgin olive oil
3 tablespoons red wine vinegar	Crusty bread to serve

DIRECTIONS

1. Heat 3 tablespoons of olive oil in a casserole dish over medium heat. Season the rabbit well and fry in batches until golden brown. Set aside.
2. Fry the onion with a pinch of salt till it's translucent. Add the garlic and chili flakes and cook for another minute.
3. Stir in the tomato purée; add the rabbit back to the pan with the wine, chicken stock, red wine vinegar, bay leaves and thyme. Bring to a boil, then cover with a lid and simmer for 1 hour.
4. Add the cherry tomatoes and cook uncovered another 30 minutes until the meat is tender.
5. Mix the parsley, garlic, lemon zest and juice with the olive oil and season to make the gremolata.
6. Serve the rabbit stew with gremolata and crusty bread

Greek Rabbit Stew (Rabbit Stifado)

Stifado (stee-FAH-do) can have endless variations based just on the tomatoes and wine. Chopped tomatoes, crushed tomatoes, tomato paste. Red wine, white wine, sweet or dry. One recipe recommends the Greek sweet wine called Mavrodaphne or port.

Stifado uses a lot of olive oil, to moisten the rabbit, which is braised slowly until it is about to fall off the bone. You can pull the meat off the bone before serving or leave the pieces in the stew. The Greeks typically leave it all on the bone.

The spices give the stew zing without heat, and the tomatoes, which are a post-1492 addition, add a bit more sweetness as well as needed acidity.

You'll want either a nice Greek red wine, a lager beer, or ouzo with a glass of water as a chaser to go with this stew. Serve with crusty bread!

PREP 20 minutes   COOK 1 hour 30 minutes   SERVES 6

INGREDIENTS

2 cottontail rabbits or 1 domestic rabbit	4 large grated tomatoes or 14-ounce can of crushed tomatoes
Kosher salt	
2 medium red onions, sliced	1 cup dry red wine
5 cloves chopped garlic	1/2 cup sweet red wine
10 allspice berries	1/2 cup chicken or rabbit stock
1 cinnamon stick	1/4 cup red wine vinegar
4 bay leaves	Freshly ground black pepper
1 tablespoon dried oregano	1/4 cup olive oil
2 tablespoons tomato paste	

DIRECTIONS

1. Cut the rabbits into serving size pieces, using everything, including belly flaps, front legs, kidneys—*everything*. Salt the pieces well and set aside for 30 minutes.

2. Heat 1/4 cup olive oil in a frying pan and brown the rabbit well. When browned, move each to a heavy, lidded pot.

3. Sauté the onions 4 to 5 minutes over medium-high heat, until they begin to brown. Add the garlic and sauté for another minute. Sprinkle with salt. Do not let the garlic burn.

4. Move the onions and garlic to the lidded pot and toss the bay leaves, oregano, allspice berries and cinnamon stick in on top.

5. Cut the tomatoes in half and run them through a coarse grater to remove skins.

6. Put the wine, sweet wine, vinegar, stock, tomato paste and grated tomatoes into the frying pan. Cook this down over high heat for 3 to 4 minutes, then pour over everything in the pot.

7. Cover the pot and bring to a simmer. Simmer for 1 hour, and check. If the rabbit is almost falling off the bone, it's ready. If not, keep simmering!

8. Grind some black pepper and drizzle some really good olive oil over everything right when you serve.

9. Serve with crusty bread or rice.

Tips:

1. Brown the rabbit really well. It makes a difference in the finished stew.

2. Use a sweet wine (Mavrodaphne if you can find it), as well as allspice and cinnamon. If you can't find Greek Mavrodaphne, use Port or any sweet red wine.

3. Like many stews, this one is best a day or two after you make it. It will keep a week in the fridge.

Old Fashioned Rabbit Stew

PREP less than 30 minutes   COOK 2+ hours   SERVES 5-6

INGREDIENTS

3 tablespoons plain flour	6 pieces of bacon, cut into ¾ in squares
2 teaspoons dried thyme,	2 onions, chopped
or 2 tablespoons chopped fresh thyme leaves	17 ounces dry cider
Sea salt and freshly ground black pepper	10 ounces chicken or vegetable stock
1/2 ounce butter	2 bay leaves
2-3 tablespoons sunflower oil	12 ounces chantenay carrots, peeled
1 large rabbit, cut into 8 pieces	5 oz frozen peas

I first saw the Three Hares design in a window in the Cathedral at Paderdorn, Germany. It is believed, in Christianity, to represent the Trinity. Its origins are unclear, however, as historians, archaeologists and researchers have found this symbol all over the world, not only in numerous Christian settings, but also in Buddhist, Islamic, Celtic, pagan, and Jewish cultures. The symbol has even been found on the walls of caves in China.

The image contains an intriguing paradox: each rabbit appears to have two ears—yet there are only three ears total.

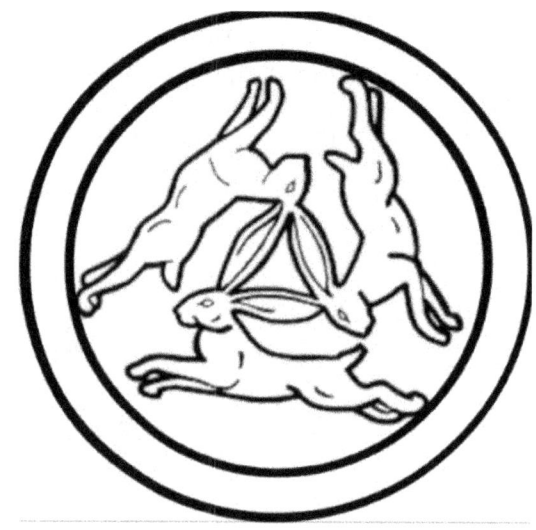

DIRECTIONS

1. Preheat the oven to 340 F.

2. Put flour, thyme, a pinch of salt and lots of freshly ground black pepper in a large Ziploc bag. Put a few rabbit pieces at a time into the bag and shake it well. This is best done with *Dancing Queen* playing at high volume. Set the coated rabbit aside.

3. Melt the butter and one tablespoon of oil in a large heavy frying pan over medium heat. Fry a few pieces of rabbit at a time, until golden-brown all over. Put the front and rear leg portions in a casserole dish.

4. Move the saddle pieces to a plate, cover loosely and set aside (these will need less cooking time, so can be added later on).

5. Add more oil to the pan and cook the bacon until the fat is browned and beginning to crisp. Add the bacon to the casserole dish.

6. Add a bit more oil to the frying pan and fry the onion 5-7 minutes, until lightly browned and beginning to soften. Add the onions to the casserole, sprinkle it with any flour still in the freezer bag and stir well.

7. Pour half of the cider into the frying pan. Stir briskly with a wooden spoon to lift any remaining food from the bottom. Simmer for a few seconds then pour into the casserole. Add the rest of the cider and the stock. Stir the bay leaves into the casserole, cover with a lid and cook in the middle of the oven for 45 minutes.

8. Remove the casserole from the oven, add the saddle pieces and carrots, turn all the rabbit portions, making sure as much of the meat is covered by liquid as possible. Return it to the oven for another 1-2 hours.

9. After the first hour, check the rabbit. It's ready when the meat is starting to fall off the bone. Stick the leg portions and the saddle pieces with a knife and if it doesn't slide in easily, return the casserole to the oven. Check again for tenderness and turn the rabbit portions every 30 minutes.

10. When the rabbit is tender, skim off any fat that has risen to the top of the casserole with a large spoon. Move the casserole to the stove. Bring to a fast simmer and cook for 3-5 minutes, or until the liquid reduces to a slightly thickened, gravy-like consistency. Stir in the frozen peas and simmer for another three minutes. Season with salt and freshly ground black pepper and serve.

Rabbit Stew with Mushrooms

Use as many types of fresh mushrooms as you can. Most grocery stores will have several kinds. The more kinds, the better. Dried porcini mushrooms add a lot to the flavor, as does the water they soaked in. Strain that water with a paper towel or coffee filter to remove dirt or grit.

An option for this recipe is to brown the whole rabbit, and put it into the stew whole. Remove it later and pick off the meat. An optional but well worth it is a liver thickener that will enrich your sauce. To go halfway with this step, mix in a large dollop of crème fraiche or sour cream in at the end.

PREP 45 minutes   COOK 1 hour 45 minutes   SERVES 4

INGREDIENTS

1 ounce dried porcini mushrooms	1 cup sherry or white wine
2 heads of garlic	1 to 2 cups mushroom soaking water
1 tablespoon extra virgin olive oil	3 cups chicken stock
1 1/2 pounds mixed mushrooms	1 tablespoon fresh thyme or 2 teaspoons dried
4 tablespoons unsalted butter	1 large parsnip
1 rabbit	Salt
3 large shallots, chopped	2 tablespoons chopped fresh parsley

DIRECTIONS

1. Preheat the oven to 375°F
2. Peel and chop the parsnip into large pieces.
3. Roast the garlic Slice the top third off the heads of garlic and drizzle the olive oil over them. Wrap the heads loosely in foil and bake for 45 minutes to an hour, or until cloves are soft and brown. Set aside to cool.
4. Soak the dried porcini mushrooms in 2 cups of hot water.
5. Cut the rabbit into pieces and sprinkle with salt. Let sit at room temperature for 30 minutes as the garlic finishes roasting. Use all of the rabbit. You can remove the ribs and other parts that have little meat on them later; they will add lots of flavor to your stew.
6. The crème fraiche-liver thickener is optional. To make it, mince the liver finely and put it in a small bowl. Whip in about 1 1/2 tablespoons crème fraiche or sour cream. Put the thickener into

a fine-meshed sieve over a bowl and push it through with a rubber spatula. Put it in the fridge to chill.

7. Chop off the tough ends of the mushroom stems. Toss them or save them for stock. Slice the mushrooms and set aside. Dice the rehydrated porcini. Pour the porcini soaking water through a paper towel into another bowl. Save the liquid.

8. Dry sauté the mushrooms. Heat a thick-bottomed large pot on high for 1 minute. Add the mushrooms and shake the pot. Stir continuously to dry sauté the mushrooms until they release their water.

9. Turn the heat down to medium-high. Scrape any mushroom bits off the bottom of the pan with a wooden spoon. Salt the mushrooms lightly. When the mushroom liquid is mostly gone, remove them to a bowl.

10. Add butter to the pot. When it melts, turn the heat down to medium. Pat the rabbit pieces dry and place in the pan. Work in batches so as not to overcrowd the pan. Brown the pieces well on all sides. Remove the rabbit pieces from the pot and set aside.

11. Sauté the shallots: Increase the heat to medium-high and add the shallots to the pot. Sauté until they wilt, about 3 minutes. Stir from time to time. Sprinkle salt on everything.

12. While the shallots are cooking, squeeze the roasted garlic into the strained mushroom soaking water. Whisk it together.

13. Add the sherry or white wine to the shallots in the pot. Use a wooden spoon to scrape off browned bits on the bottom of the pot. Let the sherry boil down by half. Add the mushroom-roasted garlic mixture and the stock. Stir to combine.

14. Add the thyme, mushrooms, rabbit, and parsnips; bring to a simmer.

15. Add the thyme, all the mushrooms, rabbit, and parsnips and bring everything to a bare simmer.

16. Simmer for 90 minutes. You want the meat to be close to falling off the bone. If you want, you can fish out all the rabbit pieces and pull the meat off the bone – it makes the dish less attractive, but it will be easier to eat. Taste for salt right before you serve and add if needed. Stir in the parsley.

17. Add the liver mixture (optional): If you are using the crème fraiche-liver mixture to thicken your stew, turn off the heat. When the stew stops bubbling, add the mixture and let it heat through for a minute before serving.

18. Do not allow the stew to boil once the liver-crème fraiche mixture is in it or it will curdle.

19. Serve with a crusty loaf of bread, a green salad, and either a hearty white wine, a dry rose, or a light red wine.

Crock Pot Rabbit Chili

PREP 15 minutes   COOK hours   SERVES 6

INGREDIENTS

3 pounds of rabbit (about 1 rabbit)	4-6 diced red peppers
Flour	1 teaspoon. cumin seed
Oil	1 teaspoon ground cumin seed
1 onion, chopped	1/2 ounce cooking chocolate, unsweetened
2 large dollops of tomato paste	3 tablespoon chili powder
1 1/2 tins of chopped tomatoes	1 teaspoon of chili flakes
a handful of fresh basil & parsley	2 pounds red kidney beans
2 teaspoons oregano	Water
2 cloves garlic paste	2 dashes of balsamic vinegar

DIRECTIONS

1. Brown rabbit and onions in oil. Add flour.
2. Stick it in the slow cooker and add everything else!
3. Slow cook for hours.

To the Chinese, the rabbit is a symbol of good luck, representing peace and tranquility. Those born in the year of the rabbit are believed to be open, optimistic, and imaginative.

White Rabbit Chili

INGREDIENTS

2 cups cubed rabbit meat	3 1/2 cups chicken broth
1 tablespoon extra virgin olive oil	4 ounces (1 can) diced green chilies
1 onion, diced	1 jalapeno pepper, de-seeded and minced
3 cloves garlic, minced	43.5 ounces (3 cans) great northern beans
1 1/2 teaspoon cumin	1/2 teaspoon salt
1/4 teaspoon cayenne pepper	1/4 teaspoon freshly ground black pepper
1 teaspoon oregano	1/4 teaspoon white pepper
3 tablespoons flour	

Topping: shredded Monterrey jack or white cheddar cheese

DIRECTIONS

1. Heat the olive oil over medium heat in a Dutch oven. Toss in the rabbit and cook until it is opaque. Scoop the rabbit out with a slotted spoon and set it aside.
2. Drop onion & garlic into the drippings. When they are tender and golden, reduce heat to low and sprinkle in the flour, stirring to coat.
3. Stir cayenne pepper, cumin, and oregano into the onions and garlic.
4. Rinse and drain the beans.
5. Pour in chicken broth, green chilies, jalapeño, beans, rabbit, salt, and peppers.
6. Bring the soup to a boil, reduce the heat and cook for another 15-20 minutes, or until the rabbit is cooked through and tender.
7. Serve topped with the shredded cheese

A Dutch oven, contrary to its name, is not an oven and does not speak Dutch. It's a heavy, wide pot with a tight-fitting lid, usually made of enameled cast iron and with handles.

STUFFED

Rabbit Saddle with Ham and Mushrooms

INGREDIENTS

1 rabbit saddle, de-boned	*Sauce*
1/4 preserved lemon, pith removed	1 carrot, chopped
6 slices parma ham	1 stick celery, chopped
4 ounces button mushrooms	1 shallot, finely sliced
1/2 cup chorizo	1 clove garlic, chopped
1-1/2 cups spinach	1 sprig thyme
1 banana shallot, finely diced	1 bay leaf
2 medium carrots	1/2 cup brandy, or cognac
1-1/2 cups new potatoes	1/2 cup double cream
1 small handful wild herbs, optional	2 teaspoons wholegrain mustard
Sea salt	Reserved rabbit bones, chopped
Freshly cracked black pepper	
Rapeseed oil, for cooking	
2 cloves garlic, finely chopped	

DIRECTIONS

1. Preheat oven to 355 F

2. Preparing the sauce will take about two hours. Place a large heavy pan over high heat. Add 2 tablespoons of rapeseed oil. When the oil is hot (about 30 seconds), add the chopped rabbit bones and stir occasionally, until they are a golden brown. Remove the bones from the pan and set aside. Add carrots, celery, onion, garlic, thyme and bay. Add a pinch of salt and cook for about 5 minutes until the vegetables are soft and caramelized residue on the bottom of the pan comes loose.

3. Add the brandy, and boil down to a syrup. Add enough water to cover the bones, and bring to a boil. Simmer for 2 hours, topping up with water when necessary to make sure the bones are covered. Strain the sauce through a fine sieve into another pan, add the cream, and boil until reduced to a thick sauce consistency. Stir in the mustard.

4. While the sauce is simmering, place a large sauté pan over medium-high heat and add 2 tablespoons of rapeseed oil. When the oil is hot, add the spinach with a pinch of salt and cook until it's wilted. Water will be released from the spinach. Move it to a colander and set aside to cool.

5. Dice the mushrooms and chorizo into small pieces. Chop the lemon.

6. Heat a large pan over high heat and add 2 tablespoons of rapeseed oil. When the oil is hot, add the diced mushrooms. Cook for a few minutes, stirring occasionally, until the mushrooms are half-cooked. Add shallots and garlic with a pinch of salt and continue cooking. After 3 minutes reduce heat to medium and add the diced chorizo. Cook for 3 more minutes, then move to a large mixing bowl and leave to cool.

7. When the spinach is cool, squeeze out the excess liquid. Then roughly chop it and add to the mushroom mix. Add diced lemon and salt and pepper to taste. This is the saddle stuffing.

8. To stuff the rabbit saddles, lay two pieces of parma ham side by side lengthwise on a chopping board. It should be about the same surface area as the rabbit saddle. If needed use an extra piece of parma ham to make sure you have enough to wrap your saddle completely. Lay the saddle skin side down on the ham and lightly season with salt and pepper. Stuff the cavity with the mushroom and spinach mix. A cylinder of mix should run through the center of the loin about half an inch wide. Pull over the parma ham to allow you to wrap your stuffed saddle into a roll. Tie it with twine using a butchers knot.

9. Boil the potatoes.

10. Cut the carrots into medium chunks to roast in the oven.

11. Heat a heavy frying pan over high heat and add 2 tablespoons of rapeseed oil. When the oil is hot, add the rabbit saddle and fry until lightly caramelized on all sides. Place in the oven for 6 minutes. Check that it is cooked in the center using either a thin skewer or temperature probe (it should be 140 F). If it needs longer, turn it over and return to the oven. When it is cooked, remove from the pan and rest on a rack for 6 minutes before untying the string and carving each into three pieces. Serve with the carrots and potatoes and a drizzle of sauce on top. Garnish with fresh herbs.

Stuffed Rabbit Roulade with Boudin

INGREDIENTS

2-3 rabbits	1/2 cup cooked rice
6 oz smoked Boudin*	3 cloves of garlic, minced
1 small diced red bell pepper	1/4 cup chopped scallions
1 small diced yellow onion	1 tablespoon crystal hot sauce
2 small diced celery stalks	1 teaspoon Worcestershire
3 sprigs thyme	1 pound pork caul fat

* Boudin is cooked sausage made from pork and rice, vegetables & seasoning

Braise

4 rabbit forelegs	4-5 springs thyme
2 medium yellow onions, medium diced	Black peppercorns
1 medium carrot diced	1 tablespoon tomato paste
1 medium celery stalk diced	1 cup dry white wine
2 bay leaves	1 quart chicken stock to cover

DIRECTIONS

Butchery

Place the rabbit bone side down on a cutting board. Pull the forearms forward. Cut behind the shoulders to remove each forearm. Remove the hind legs by cutting toward the hip joint and popping the leg out of its socket creating a visible path for your knife and easy removal. Saddle: Begin by cutting an incision on both sides of the vertebrae starting at the hind quarters working your way towards the neck of the rabbit. Using a paring knife, angle the blade against the ribs and carefully fillet along the ribs away from the vertebrae as if you were filleting a fish. Once the saddle and the rib cage are no longer intact, simply cut straight down alongside the backbone to remove the remaining tenderloin from the hind sockets.

Braise the forelegs for the roulade stuffing

1. Caramelize the forelegs in a hot saute pan. When it's golden brown, remove and set aside. Immediately add onions, carrot and celery to the same pan and cook until lightly golden. Add tomato paste and cook for 2 more minutes. Deglaze with white wine, scraping the caramelized bits from the bottom of the pan to keep all flavors. Add the legs back to the pan, cover with parchment paper or aluminum foil and place in a 325 degree oven for 90 minutes. The braised rabbit should fall right off the bone when finished.

2. Strain liquid from the pan through a fine-mesh sieve into a small sauce pot. Wait 5 minutes and skim the surface of the braising liquid extracting any visible fat. Place on medium-low flame and reduce to a sauce consistency. This is rabbit jus.

Stuffing

1. Pick the forelegs of all meat (being careful not to include any bones) and place in a bowl.

2. Remove the Boudin from its casing and add to the rabbit meat.

3. Sweat the onion, celery, and bell pepper in a sauté pan until soft. Add garlic, thyme, and parsley and continue cooking 3-4 minutes. Add to the rabbit mixture along with the remaining ingredients. Season the stuffing to taste with salt and pepper. If stuffing gets dry add some of the braising liquid.

Rolling the Roulade

1. Lay each saddle out flat, skin side down. Season each saddle with salt.

2. Spread the stuffing evenly; hugging the tenderloin (or meatier) side of the saddle. Roll the saddle tightly into an even roulade.

3. Take the caul fat out and lay if flat on a cutting board. Cut the caul fat appropriately so that each roulade may receive to full layers of fat. Place the roulade at the base of the cut caul fat and roll as if you were rolling cigar. This will aid in moisture retention.

Stuffed Rabbit with Chorizo and Scallops

PREP 2+ hours   COOK 10-15 minutes   SERVES

INGREDIENTS

Rabbit:	*Scallops*
2 rabbit saddles with livers	12 large scallops or 20 small scallops
1-1/2 cups Spanish chorizo	2 teaspoons rapeseed oil
1/4 onion	2 knobs of butter
Rapeseed oil	Sea salt
Dill, chervil, alfalfa sprouts of other herb	Sweetcorn
Extra virgin olive oil	1-1/2 canned sweetcorn kernels, drained
	3-1/2 tablespoonsdouble cream
	1/2 cup chicken stock
	1 fresh corn on the cob, in husk
	1 teaspoon rapeseed oil

DIRECTIONS

1. Chop the onion very finely. Skin and chop the chorizo.
2. Sauté onion in rapeseed oil until translucent. Remove onions from the pan and let cool.
3. Remove the loins from each rabbit saddle and belly flap and the fillets from underneath. Leave the liver if it's attached. Trim the silver skin membrane.
4. Remove fat from the belly flaps, prick them with a knife and cover them with parchment paper or cling film. Beat them with a rolling pin to tenderize and flatten them.
5. When the onions are cool (are we talking 60s cool or 90s cool?), blend them in a blender with the chorizo.
6. Lay two pieces of cling film on the counter and smooth them down with a damp cloth. Lay a flattened belly flap onto each. Lay a loin down the length of it. Take one quarter of the stuffing and shape it into a sausage, laying it beside the loin. Slice the liver into lengths and lay it on top of the stuffing.
7. Roll the film over each loin, wrapping the belly around the loin and stuffing, making sure the film is tight. Tie the ends. Roll all loins. Chill in the refrigerator for an hour.

8. While the rabbit chills, bring the cream and stock to a boil. Pour them into the blender with the sweetcorn and blend until smooth. Pass the mixture through a fine sieve. Season with salt, pepper, dill, thyme, or any herbs. Put this in a container and cover it with cling film that touches the surface. Chill in the refrigerator.

9. Cook the whole sweetcorn in salted boiling water, in its husk if you can for 15 minutes, until tender. Then chill in the refrigerator.

10. When the corn is chilled, remove the husk. Cut the kernels off, keeping them connected in large pieces if possible. Set aside. Char these before serving them.

11. Remove the cling from the chilled rabbit. It should hold its shape. Lay out four more pieces of cling film. Place four slices of pancetta vertically on each. They should overlap each other a little. Set the rolled rabbit horizontally on top and wrap it up so that the pancetta is wrapped around the rabbit. Tie the ends and put in the refrigerator for another hour.

12. When the rabbit is chilled add 2 tablespoons of rapeseed oil to a large nonstick frying pan. Set on medium heat. Remove the rabbit rolls from the film and set them in the pan, seam-side down. Cook 10-15 minutes, turning often for even cooking and even color. When the core temperature is 140-147 F, remove the rabbit rolls from the pan and put them in a warm place.

13. At 10 minutes into cooking the rabbit rolls, start the scallops. Put a large non-stick frying pan over high heat and add oil. When it's hot, put the scallops in. In about three minutes, flip them all over.

14. Add butter. When it foams, baste the scallops for one minute. Remove them from the pan, season them and set them aside in a warm place.

15. Char the sweet corn in a hot pan with a dash of oil.

16. Spoon the chilled sweet corn sauce onto each plate. Carve the rabbit rolls into three and set them on top. Add a few scallops to each plate and a piece of charred corn. Place herbs on top and drizzle it all with a bit of olive oil

Stuffed Rabbit with Mushrooms, Spinach, and Cheese

INGREDIENTS

2 boneless rabbit loins (saddles)	2 finely minced shallots
1/2 pound mushrooms	1 package fresh spinach leaves,
2 ounces goat cheese,	4 slices sliced proscuitto,
3-4 garlic cloves	3 tablespoons olive oil
Port wine (or whatever is open)	

DIRECTIONS

1. Chop half the mushrooms and slice half. Chop spinach leaves. Roast 2 garlic cloves, mince 2.
2. Trim rabbit saddles and cut in half down the middle. Lightly pound them between two sheets of parchment paper with a mallet to even out thickness to 1/2 to 3/4 inch thick.
3. Sauté chopped mushrooms and shallot with 1 tablespoon of oil until soft. Stir in port and reduce. Salt and pepper to taste. Remove from pan. Add spinach to pan. Sauté until wilted. Add in rosemary or thyme if desired.
4. Mix goat cheese and roasted garlic with a fork.
5. Put a slice of proscuitto on each section of rabbit; top with a spoonful of sauteed mushrooms and dot with the goat cheese mixture. Roll it up and place seam side down on clean plate. Cover with plastic wrap and chill in refrigerator for at least 15 minutes.
6. Heat 2 tablespoons of olive oil in an oven safe skillet on medium high. Preheat oven to 325 F.
7. Put panko, flour, and eggs in separate shallow bowls. Dip rabbit rolls in flour, egg and then roll in panko. Brown rabbit on each side (1 -2 minutes), then put skillet in oven to finish. Bake 10-13 minutes until done.
8. While rabbit is baking, sauté sliced mushrooms in a skillet until they begin to release water and wilt, add a bit of wine and cherry tomatoes. Season well with salt and fresh pepper and simmer.
9. Remove rabbit from oven and set on platter. Serve with sautéed mushrooms and potatoes.

PASTA

Like chicken, beef, shrimp or any other meat, rabbit can be combined with any kind of pasta. Take the following recipes as jumping-off points (it's what rabbits do best!) and have fun!

Pulled Rabbit and Morel Ravioli

INGREDIENTS

2 tablespoons sweet paprika	3/4 cups morels, chopped
3 tablespoons dark chocolate, grated	Zest and juice of 1 lemon
1/4 cup soft brown sugar	1/8 cup wild garlic, ripped into shreds
1 garlic clove, crushed	*Ravioli*
2 tablespoons white wine vinegar	3-1/4 cups plain flour. extra for dusting
4 tablespoons olive oil	3 large eggs, beaten
1-1/4 cups sweet cider	1 tablespoon crushed pink peppercorns
1 rabbit, skinned and gutted	Sea salt

DIRECTIONS

1. Preheat oven to 300 F.
2. Mix together paprika, chocolate, sugar, garlic, vinegar and 2 tablespoons of olive oil in a large bowl and coat the rabbit in it.
3. Set the rabbit in a roasting pan filled with the cider. Cover with foil and cook for 3 hours, basting every hour.
4. Remove the foil and turn the oven to 280 F. Cook for a further 2 hours.
5. Remove the rabbit, use two forks to shred the meat and remove the bones.
6. Put 1 tablespoon of oil in a pan and fry the morel mushrooms 2-3 minutes until soft, then add half the lemon juice and half the wild garlic. (None of that quiet, rule-following garlic! Party hearty!) Stir, then add to the bowl of rabbit meat. Mix well.
7. Place the flour in a large bowl and make a well in the middle. Pour the eggs into the well.
8. Whisk the flour and egg together. When well-mixed, shape it into a ball and knead for 10 minutes. Divide the dough into four. Wrap each in clear film. Chill for 5 minutes.
9. On a floured surface, roll out one of the balls into a rectangle about 8x11" so it is extremely thin. Cut it into four equal strips with a sharp knife or ravioli wheel.
10. Dot five teaspoons of the rabbit-morel mix along two of the strips. Brush cold water on the pasta around the filling. Lay the other strips of the pasta carefully on top and press down to seal

around the edges and between the filling. Cut between the filling to make 5 ravioli. Chill, divided by clear film. Repeat with the other 3 pasta balls for a total of 20.

11. Cook the ravioli in batches in boiling water for 5–6 minutes each. Replace the water for each batch. In a frying pan, heat a tablespoon of oil and add the wild garlic, lemon zest and remaining juice. Stir-fry for 1 minute.

12. Coat the pasta with the olive oil mixture and season with salt and crushed peppercorns, then serve on warmed plates.

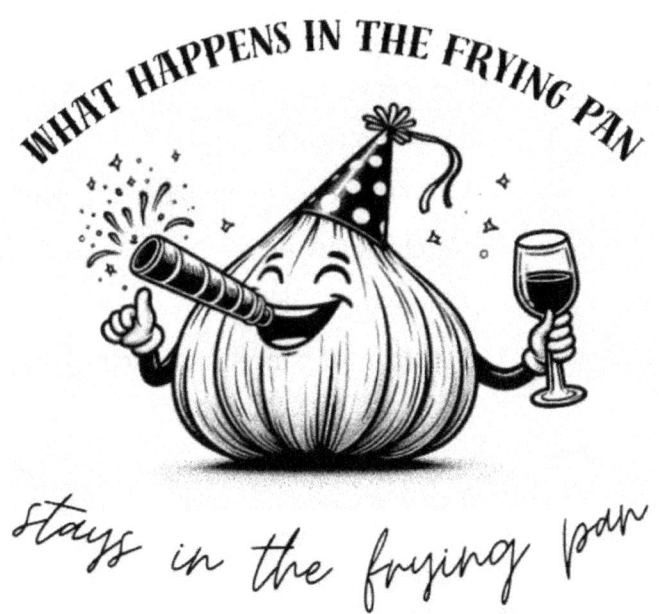

Confit of Rabbit and Green Olive in Saffron Tortellini

PREP 1 hour   COOK overnight + 20 minutes   SERVES 10

INGREDIENTS

Confit rabbit and green olive filling	*Pasta Dough*
1 medium sized rabbit	4 sachets saffron
1-1/4 cups extra virgin olive oil	1 cup boiling water
3-4 star anise	2 cups flour
6 whole peppercorns	Pinch of salt
1/2 cup green table olives	2 tablespoons extra virgin olive oil
1/4 cup cream	7 egg yolks

Sauce	*Accompaniments*
7 ounces butter	1 cup fresh peas (shelled and peeled)
1 cup cream	1/4 cup snow peas
reserved saffron water (above)	4 large tomatoes
	6-8 strips of pancetta or bacon

DIRECTIONS

Filling

1. Clean the rabbit, remove any excess pieces of fat and remove the head.
2. If you have a pizza oven or wood fire oven, roast the rabbit for 30 minutes over an open flame for extra flavor. If not, put the rabbit in a cast iron pot and cover it with the olive oil and spices. Bake overnight at 160° F.
3. In the morning, let the oil cool slightly and remove the rabbit. Shred the meat off the bone.
4. Remove the pits from the green olives and chop them finely. Add them to the rabbit and drizzle just enough cream over it all to bind. Season well with salt and pepper.

Pasta dough

1. When the rabbit goes in the oven for the night, soak the saffron in boiling water in a small bowl, cover it with cling film and leave it overnight. In the morning, reduce the saffron to just over a 1/2 cup in a small saucepan.

2. Pour flour and salt into a large bowl. Make a well in the center, add olive oil, 1/4 cup of the saffron water, and egg yolks. Knead it into dough until it's smooth and silky. Wrap in cling film and put it in the refrigerator for 10 minutes.

3. Use a pasta machine or rolling pin to roll the chilled dough into thin sheets. Use a round cookie cutter or glass of about 3 inches to stamp out circles of dough.

4. Spoon a small teaspoon of filling into the center of each circle, brush the edges of the dough with water or egg wash, fold over and seal tightly. Bring the edges back around and seal together.

5. Keep the tortellini covered in the refrigerator until you are ready to blanch them in boiling water for about 3 minutes, or until al dente and serve immediately.

Sauce

1. Melt the butter in a saucepan. Let it bubble until it's a golden brown but not burned.

2. Whisk in the cream and the rest of the saffron liquid. Put it back on the stove and reduce it to coating consistency.

Accompaniments

1. Peel the peas and blanch* them and refresh.

2. Slice the snow peas at an angle and blanch them.

3. Blanch the tomatoes, and cut them into small cubes.

4. Toss all the vegetables together and drizzle with extra virgin olive oil.

5. Fry the bacon or pancetta until it's crispy.

* Blanching means putting food into boiling water briefly, then moving it to a bowl of ice water

To Serve
1. Blanch the tortellini and toss in olive oil
2. Put a spoonful of the vegetables in the middle of the plate. Place 3 tortellini on top and arrange the bacon or pancetta around the pasta.
3. With an electric handheld blender, froth the sauce just a bit and drizzle it over the pasta and around the plate.
4. Garnish with pea shoots.

There is an old Cornish legend that a maiden who has loved greatly and been betrayed, dies of a broken heart or from another cause related to the betrayal or unfaithfulness of her loved one, she will return as a white hare. She will haunt her beloved, mostly seen by him but sometimes by others, too. She may save him from dangers for a time, but she will ultimately cause his death. One such story was recorded in Robert Hunt's book *The drolls, traditions and superstitions of Old Cornwall*, published in 1860.

The moral of the story is: If you're going to be an unfaithful cad, don't do it in Cornwall!

Rabbit Meatballs with Porcini Tagliatelle

This recipe uses the porcini rabbit from the recipe in the BRAISED section.

INGREDIENTS

1 8.8 oz package Morelli Porcini Mushroom Tagliatelle	1 egg yolk
Leftover braising liquid from Porcini Braised Rabbit	2 eggs
Rabbit legs	3 tablespoons mayonnaise
2 tablespoons minced flat leaf parsley	1 tablespoon Canola oil
Extra parsley for garnish	1/2 cup minced onion, caramelized
1 teaspoon lemon juice	1 teaspoon minced fresh thyme
1/4 cup of heavy cream	1 teaspoon lemon juice
1 tablespoon Unsalted Butter	8 Porcini Braised Rabbit Legs
	4 rabbit kidneys, minced (optional)
Meatballs:	1-1/2 ounces dried Porcinis
1 cup Panko Bread Crumbs	Salt to taste

DIRECTIONS

1. Rehydrate the Porcinis and mince them finely. Pull the meat off rabbit legs. Shred and mince it finely. Mix all meatball ingredients together in a large bowl. Shape into meatballs.

2. Simmer the Porcini braising liquid down to about a cup.

3. Bring a pot of salted water to a boil.

4. Sear the meatballs in a hot, oiled skillet until well-browned.

5. Reduce the heat under the pan to low and add the reduced braising liquid and cream to the meatballs. Bring it to a simmer, then remove it from the heat. Periodically baste the meatballs while waiting for the pasta.

6. Boil the pasta until it's just a bit tougher than al dente. Remove it from the water and add it to the skillet with the meatballs.

7. Add parsley and toss it all to coat everything. Squeeze in the remaining lemon juice, toss again and sprinkle parsley on top.

Rabbit Agnolotti Pasta

INGREDIENTS

Pasta

3 cups of semolina flour

4 large eggs

1 teaspoon salt

Filling

1 whole rabbit cut into pieces, on the bone

1/4 cup carrot, diced

1/4 cup celery, diced

1/2 cup onion, diced

2 cloves garlic, chopped

2 4" branches of fresh rosemary

6 fresh sage leaves

1 dried bay leaf

1 cup dry white wine like Orvieto

1/3 cup grated Parmigiano Reggiano

1/3 cup fresh ricotta

1 egg

1 tablespoon fresh rosemary, chopped

1/2 tablespoons fresh sage, chopped

Salt and pepper

1/4 cup butter

8 or 10 sage leaves (chopped) to serve

more Parmigiano

DIRECTIONS

Pasta

1. Put the flour in a bowl and make a well in the middle. Pour the beaten egg and salt into the well. With a fork, mix the flour into the egg.

2. Knead the dough on a well-floured board for 3 or 4 minutes until it's smooth and firm.

3. Wrap the dough in plastic and chill it in the fridge for 20-30 minutes.

Filling

1. Season the rabbit pieces on all sides with salt and pepper.

2. Add olive oil to a large heavy pot. Brown the rabbit in batches to avoid crowding, then set aside.

3. Add the carrot, onion and celery to the pot and sauté until they're soft and just starting to color.

4. Add the garlic and cook for a minute. Return the rabbit to the pot, with any accumulated juices.

5. Add the fresh herbs and wine and enough water to come half way up the sides of the rabbit pieces. Put the lid on and cook over low heat for about an hour and a half until the meat is tender.

6. Remove it from the pot and set aside to cool.

7. Continue cooking the sauce over medium heat, reducing it down to a syrup. While the sauce is reducing, take all the meat from the bones and chop it finely.

8. Place the cool meat in a bowl. Mix in the Parmigiano, ricotta, egg and chopped herbs.

9. When the sauce cools, push it through a fine sieve, including the vegetables. Scrape the strained vegetables off the back of the sieve and adding them to the filling with the reduction.

10. Season to taste with salt and pepper as needed. Refrigerate until needed.

Agnolotti

1. Roll out a small piece of pasta dough using a pasta maker or rolling pin, with plenty of flour, until it is very thin, into a long rectangle about 3 inches wide.

2. Place 2 teaspoon dots of cold filling about an inch apart along the length of the pasta. Brush a little water on the dough around the filling to help it stick and then fold the dough in half over the filling.

3. Squeeze out the air around the filling and then cut out your agnolotti, crimping the edges and sealing them shut. Repeat until all are finished. Set the agnolotti on a floured baking sheet lined with wax paper and refrigerate or freeze until needed.

4. To finish, drop the agnolotti into a large pot of well-salted boiling water.

5. Melt the butter over medium heat in a large pan. When it stops sizzling, add the chopped sage.

6. When the agnolotti floats to the top of the water, let it cook for two more minutes. Use a slotted spoon to remove it to the hot sage butter.

7. Toss to coat the agnolotti in sage butter, then sprinkle it with Parmigiano.

8. Serve in a hot bowl.

Rabbit Ragu

INGREDIENTS

1/4 cup extra-virgin olive oil *(plus 1 tablespoon)*	1 medium carrot
2 tablespoons unsalted butter	1 celery rib
1/4 pound pancetta, diced	1 cup light dry red wine *(such as Pinot Noir)*
1 tablespoon fresh sage	1 (14-ounce) can Italian Plum Tomatoes
1-1/2 teaspoons fresh rosemary	1-1/4 teaspoons course gray sea salt
1 3-pounds rabbit	1/2 teaspoon coarsely ground black pepper
1 medium onion	

DIRECTIONS

1. Chop the sage, rosemary, onion, carrot, celery, and tomatoes.
2. Dice the pancetta and cube the rabbit meat into 1 inch pieces.
3. Heat oil and butter in a 12-inch heavy skillet at least 2 inches deep over medium heat.
4. Add pancetta, stirring occasionally, for 2 minutes. Add sage and rosemary, stirring, for 30 seconds.
5. Add rabbit, stirring occasionally, until rabbit is no longer pink on the outside, 2 to 3 minutes.
6. Add onion, carrot, and celery and cook, stirring occasionally, until softened, about 5 minutes.
7. Add wine and simmer, uncovered, stirring occasionally, until liquid is reduced to about 1 cup, 10 to 15 minutes.
8. Add tomatoes, sea salt, and pepper and simmer, stirring occasionally, until sauce is thickened, 5 to 10 minutes.

Tagliatelle with Rabbit in Mustard Sauce

INGREDIENTS

1 pound rabbit meat	2 tablespoons mustard
White pepper to taste	1 carrot
Salt to taste	1 onion
Flour to taste	1 or 2 cloves garlic
Plant oil to taste	1/4 cup white wine
1-1/2 cups chicken broth	1 sprig thyme
3/4 cup double cream	

DIRECTIONS

1. Preheat oven to 170 F.
2. Slice the rabbit meat finely. Season on all sides with salt and pepper and sprinkle it lightly with flour. Shake off excess. Heat oil in a saucepan and fry rabbit until golden brown, then set it in a sieve.
3. Cut carrots into thin wedges, onion into half-rings. Drain the excess oil from the pan, pour new oil and cook the onion, carrots and garlic. Fry it until transparent onion, but any remaining rabbit bits and flour must not burn. This is the base of the sauce.
4. Pour wine in the saucepan. While it's evaporating, scrape rabbit bits and flour from the bottom. Pour in the broth, return the meat to the saucepan and heat it.
5. In a separate bowl, mix cream with mustard.
6. Add the mustard cream while the pan is over medium heat and turn the heat up. At the first signs of a boil turn off the heat. Throw a sprig of thyme into the saucepan and cover it with a lid.
7. Put the saucepan into the 170 degrees oven for 40 minutes. On taking it out, remove the meat from the sauce and let the sauce evaporate to the desired consistency.
8. Start the pasta but stop cooking it 1 minute before it's done. Strain the sauce then combine it with meat and pasta. Mix until the sauce cover the tagliatelle.
9. Spread the pasta on a plate. Garnish it with carrot and thyme.

TERRINES

Terrine can refer both to a cooking vessel and to the food that is cooked or served in these pans. It is a loaf-shaped dish with layers of meat or fish, and can include vegetables. They're usually served cold or at room temperature.

Rabbit and Pork Terrine with Peppercorns

PREP 25 minutes   COOK 2 hours 15 minutes   SERVES 8

INGREDIENTS

Meat from 3 wild rabbits:	2 tablespoons butter
2-1/2 cups brown meat from the back legs and trimmings	2 garlic cloves, bruised
a bit under half from the loins	3 shallots, finely chopped
16-20 slices dry-cured streaky unsmoked bacon	A few thyme sprigs
4 ounces small pickled cucumbers, plus extra to serve	Pinch of ground allspice
1 tablespoon green peppercorns in brine, drained	3-4 tablespoons brandy
2 cups boneless pork belly, cut into chunks	Splash of vegetable oil

DIRECTIONS

1. Remove the meat from the rabbit. Chop leg meat, trimmings and pork belly finely in a processor and put in a bowl. Set the loins aside without mincing them.

2. Cook the garlic, shallots and thyme together in butter for 8 minutes or until the shallots are soft. Pour over the minced meat, add the allspice, peppercorns and 3 tablespoons brandy, then mix well. Chill for at least 1 hour in the refrigerator.

3. Add oil to the pan and brown the loins but don't need to cook them through. If desired, add 1 tablespoon brandy to the pan and flambé them to finish. Set aside on a plate and tip any pan juices into the minced mixture.

4. Heat oven to 320 F.

5. Remove the garlic from the mince. Line a loaf tin with foil. Lay the bacon crosswise in the pan, so that the ends of each piece hang over the long sides of the pan. Arrange the bacon so the base of the pan is covered with overlapping slices and they come neatly up the sides in a single layer and overhang generously. Boil water.

6. Press a third of the mince into the tin. Make a lengthways channel along one side, then press in a line of loin pieces. Scatter half the cornichons over the other side.

7. Add the next third of mince and repeat, this time with the loins and cornichons on the opposite sides. Cover with the remaining mince, then bring the bacon over the top. Wrap tightly in foil and put in a deep roasting tin. Pour in enough hot water to come halfway up the terrine and bake

for 2 hours. It's done when a skewer comes out hot from the middle of the terrine, and the juices run clear. Add to the water as needed.

8. Leave the loaf tin on a rack in a roasting tin. Tear cardboard to fit the top of the loaf tin. Add a few layers and put something heavy on top to press the terrine down. Cool to room temperature, then chill in the refrigerator, ideally overnight. Remove the weight and re-wrap the terrine in clean foil or cling film. It's not necessary but best, to let it sit for 2 days in the refrigerator before eating.

9. Serve with the pickle salad and remaining small pickles.

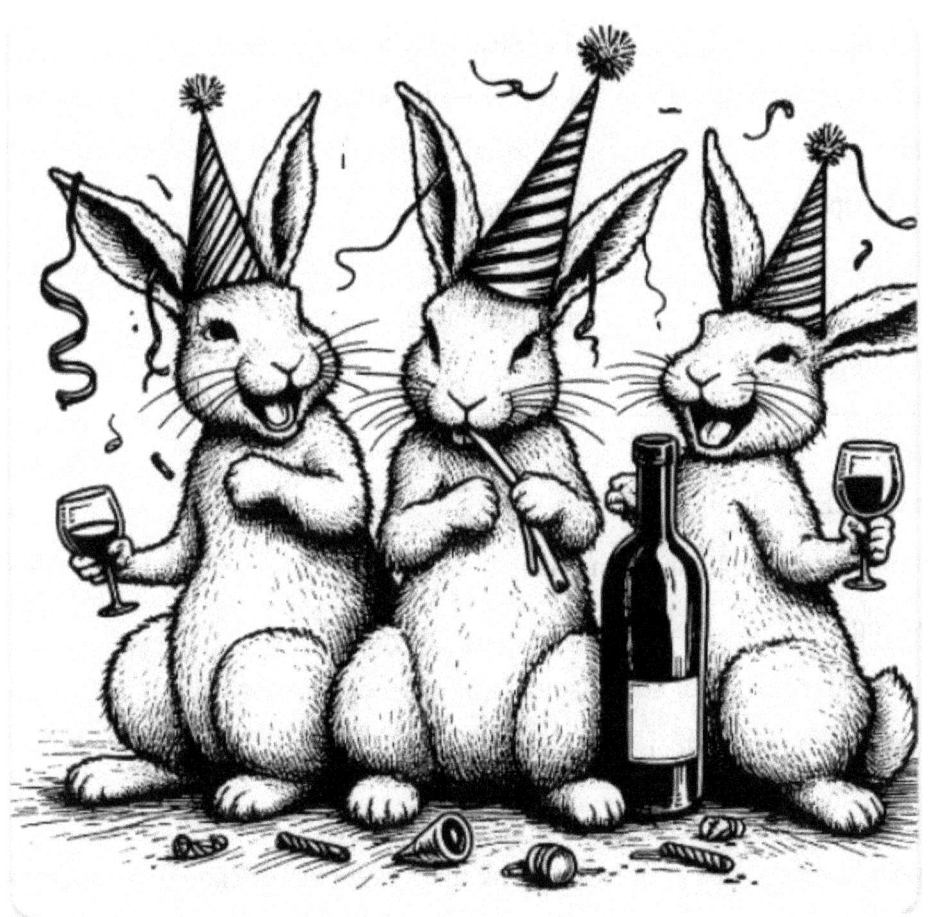

Olive and Pistachio Rabbit Terrine

PREP: 11-1/2 hours SERVES: 40 hors d'oeuvres

INGREDIENTS

1 (3-lb) rabbit, cut into 8 pieces	2 teaspoons of unflavored gelatin
4 shallots, thinly sliced	1/2 teaspoon fennel seeds
2 carrots, thinly sliced	1/2 cup brine-cured green olives
3 fresh parsley sprigs	1/3 cup salted shelled pistachios,
2 fresh thyme sprigs	3 tablespoons fresh chives
1 leek (green part only), rinsed	1 teaspoon fresh thyme
1 head garlic, unpeeled	1/2 teaspoon salt
1/2 teaspoon black peppercorns,	3/4 teaspoon black pepper
1/2 teaspoon salt	18 very thin slices firm white sandwich bread, buttered
6 1/4 cups cold water	and cut into 2
2 large egg whites plus shells	

YOU WILL ALSO NEED

- 2 tapered narrow rectangular terrine pans
- Kitchen string
- 2 11-1/2" by 1-1/2" strips of corrugated cardboard wrapped well in tin foil
- 2 rolling pins or high-shouldered wine bottles

DIRECTIONS

1. If your eggs, like ours, are farm fresh, wash them before use. Then grind them in a blender.

2. Halve the garlic heads. Crack the peppercorns. Toast the fennel seeds. Pit and coarsely chop the green olives. Shell and coarsely chop the pistachios. Slice the chives into thin strips. Chop the thyme. Save the egg shells and crush them well.

3. Remove fat, kidneys, and liver from rabbit if necessary. Put rabbit, shallots, carrots, parsley, thyme, leek, garlic, peppercorns, 1/4 teaspoon salt, and 6 cups of water in a 4-quart heavy pot and bring to a boil, skimming froth.

4. Reduce heat; simmer rabbit, partially covered, until tender, about an hour. Cool rabbit in broth, uncovered, 30 minutes. Separate rabbit meat from broth. Pour broth through a fine sieve into a bowl, discarding solids. Whisk egg whites in another bowl until foamy. Add ground egg shells. Whisk it all into a broth and pour it into a clean bowl.

5. Heat on medium, stirring and scraping the bottom constantly. When the stock begins to bubble (about 10 minutes), reduce the heat and simmer, without stirring, until all impurities rise to surface and form a crust, and broth underneath is clear, which should take another 10 minutes.

6. While broth is simmering, shred rabbit meat, not too finely. Remove all the small bones.

7. Pour the broth through a sieve lined with two layers of damp paper towels into a bowl and let all broth drain through. Discard any solids. Or feed them to your chickens. If the liquid doesn't drain completely, tap the edge of the sieve with a spoon until it does. Broth should be completely clear; if not, run it through sieve again with clean dampened paper towels.

8. Boil the clarified broth down to 2 1/2 cups. If necessary, add water to bring it up to 2-1/2 cups. Bring it to a simmer.

9. Sprinkle gelatin over 1/4 cup cold water and soften 1 minute, then whisk into hot broth until dissolved. Stir in Madeira and 1/4 teaspoon salt, or to taste.

10. Oil terrine pans and line with a sheet of plastic wrap large enough to drape over edges. Place terrines on a tray. Cut 4 18-inch pieces of kitchen string and place 2 crosswise under each terrine 2 inches from each end (they will be used to secure rolling pins or bottles to terrines).

11. Grind fennel seeds and mix into rabbit, olives, pistachios, chives, thyme, salt, and pepper in a large bowl. Divide mixture between terrine pans, then stir broth well and pour slowly into each pan, filling to 1/4 inch from top.

12. If any broth remains, cover it and chill it. Place a foil-wrapped cardboard strip on top of each terrine pan, then rest something heavy on it, creating just enough pressure to press the cardboard about 1/2 inch into terrine. Expect some broth to spill over.

13. Chill terrines on tray 3 hours, then remove string, weights, and cardboard. Heat any reserved jelled broth (including spillover on tray) until it becomes liquid and add to terrines. Cover with overhanging plastic wrap and chill at least 6 hours more.

14. To unmold terrines, unwrap plastic wrap and invert molds onto a long narrow platter, pulling slightly on plastic to release terrines from molds, then removing it. Cut terrines with a serrated knife into 1/3-inch-thick slices and serve on toasts.

Toast spices in a dry heavy skillet over moderate heat, stirring, until fragrant and a shade or two darker.
** To toast, arrange bread slices on a baking sheet and spread with 2 tablespoons butter. Toast in middle of oven until golden, about 10 minutes.

Rabbit Terrine with Bacon, Lemon and Herbs

PREP 30 minutes   COOK 1 hour 15 minutes + cooling & chilling   SERVES: 12

INGREDIENTS

2 ounces butter	1/2 teaspoon freshly grated nutmeg
3 round shallots, finely chopped	1 medium free-range egg, beaten
5-6 tbsp dry white wine	1 teaspoon salt
1-1/2 pounds boneless rabbit meat (see tip)	1/2 teaspoon ground black pepper
3/4 pound skinned and boned chicken	1/2 pound thinly sliced pancetta or bacon
1/2 pound cubed pancetta or rindless bacon	4 fresh bay leaves
Zest of 1 lemon, finely grated	Sunflower oil
2 tablespoons chopped thyme leaves	

DIRECTIONS

1. Preheat the oven to 340 F.
2. Melt butter in a pan. Add shallots, cover and cook 7-10 minutes until soft but not browned.
3. Add the wine and simmer 3-4 minutes until the wine reduces and the mixture is thick and syrupy. Set it aside till it's completely cool—as cool as the Fonz.
4. Chop the rabbit, chicken, and 1/2 pound of pancetta or bacon finely.
5. Knead the minced meats into a large mixing bowl with the shallot and wine mixture, lemon zest, thyme leaves, nutmeg, beaten egg, salt and black pepper.
6. Lay the slices of the pancetta or bacon across the bottom of a bread loaf pan. The bacon should overlap so there are no gaps and go up the sides of the pan with the ends overhanging the edges of the pan.
7. Press the terrine mixture into the corners of the dish, then fold the ends of the pancetta/bacon over to cover the mix. Extra slices may be needed on top to cover the filling.
8. Lay the bay leaves on top down the middle of the terrine.
9. Cover the terrine with an oiled sheet of foil and a lid if there is one. Set the terrine pan into a small deep roasting tin or pan, pour freshly boiled water into the roasting tin until it comes

halfway up the side of the terrine dish and set it in the oven. Cook for about 1-1/4 hours until the juices run clear when pierced in the center with a skewer.

10. Remove from the oven, remove the terrine from the roasting tin, and let it cool for an hour. Put the terrine pan into the refrigerator to chill.

11. Remove it from the pan and slice to serve.

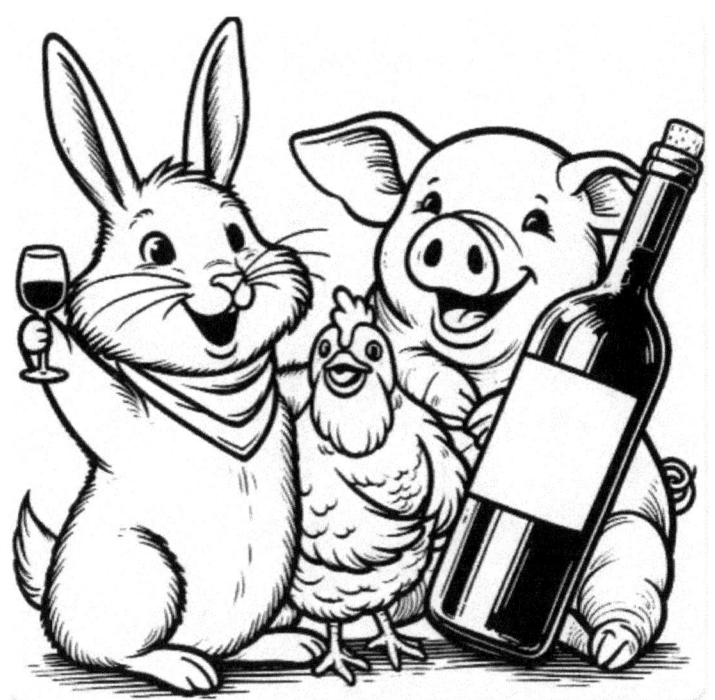

PIES, CASSEROLES

Rabbit Pie

INGREDIENTS

1 wild rabbit	Salt
8.5 cups chicken stock (or water or half and half)	Freshly ground black pepper
1 stick celery, chopped	1 quantity short crust pastry
1/2 carrot, sliced	(see recipe, right)
1 onion, chopped	1/2 cup fresh breadcrumbs
1 piece lemon zest	
1 stalk parsley	*Sauce*
1 bay leaf	3-1/2 ounces butter
1 sprig thyme	3-1/2 ounces plain flour
1 teaspoons black peppercorns	4-1/4 reserved cooking liquid
3-1/2 ounces smoked streaky bacon, minced	1/2 cup cream
7 ounces button mushrooms, sliced	Juice of 1 lemon
3-1/2 ounces flaked almonds, toasted	Salt
1 cup freshly chopped parsley	Freshly ground black pepper

DIRECTIONS

1. Preheat oven to 400 F.

2. Remove kidneys and liver from rabbit and reserve. Simmer rabbit in stock with celery, carrot, onion, zest, herbs and peppercorns until back legs test tender, 1-2 hours. Allow rabbit to cool completely in stock. Remove rabbit and set strained cooking liquid aside. Strip all meat from carcass and cut into small pieces. Discard bones.

3. Sauté bacon and mushrooms. Sear kidneys and liver, then chop and mix with rabbit, bacon, mushrooms and almonds in a bowl. Mix in parsley and season well. Cover with cling wrap.

Sauce

1. Cook butter and flour over low heat to make a roux. Slowly stir in reserved rabbit stock and bring to a simmer. Add cream and lemon juice and simmer for 10 minutes. Check seasoning, then add enough sauce to meat to make a creamy filling. Cool completely.

2. Line an 11x7x2 pan with pastry (reserve some pastry to make a latticed top) and bake for 20 minutes.

3. Remove pastry case from oven and allow to cool. Lower oven temperature to 355 F. Spoon filling into pastry case. Sprinkle breadcrumbs on top and criss-cross strips of pastry over the filling (optional). Bake 15-20 minutes until the pastry is well browned.

4. Serve with chutney or pickled fruit.

Bede tells us of a 'goddess,' Eostre from medieval England who by way of Jacob Grimm becomes entangled with the Germanic Ostara. Folklore tells us she found a bird with frozen wings and rescued it by turning it into a rabbit, which then laid beautifully colored eggs on her feast day. This is given as background for the association of rabbits and eggs with Easter.

Old English Rabbit Pie

INGREDIENTS

Suet crust pastry:	Salt
12 ounces self-rising flour	Black pepper
6 ounces shredded suet	2 medium onions, chopped fairly small
1/2 teaspoon salt	8 ounces unsmoked streaky bacon
Black pepper	1 medium cooking apple, peeled and sliced
	4 ounces pitted prunes, chopped
Filling:	1/2 pint dry cider
1 rabbit, about 3 pounds, cut into joints	3/4 pint stock or water
1-1/2 ounces plain flour	1/2 whole nutmeg, grated
1-1/2 ounces butter	1 bay leaf

DIRECTIONS

1. Pre-heat the oven to 425°F
2. Wash the rabbit joints and place them (apart from the ribs) in a large saucepan.
3. Add the onion and apple.
4. Remove the rind from the bacon, chop it into 1 inch pieces and add to the saucepan. Add the bay leaf, salt, pepper, cider and stock. Turn on the heat to medium-high. When it simmers, skim off any scum that rises, lower the heat, put a lid on and let it simmer on low for an hour, until tender.
5. Use a slotted spoon to move rabbit, bacon, apple and onion to the pie dish. Toss in chopped prunes. If you're not that great an aim, consider just setting them down and stirring them in.
6. Mix the flour and butter to a smooth paste, then drop it, in peanut-sized pieces, into the stock in the saucepan. Stir over medium heat to melt and thicken the sauce. Sprinkle in nutmeg. When the sauce begins to simmer, pour it over the rabbit.

Suet Crust Pastry

1. Mix together flour, salt, pepper and suet. Add enough cold water to form a soft, elastic dough that leaves the bowl cleanly.

2. Roll the dough out to an inch wider than the top of the pie plate, and cut off a 1 inch strip all around. Dampen the edge of the pie plate and press this strip around the rim of the plate. Next, dampen the rim of the pastry, and set the round pastry on top, crimping all round to seal the edge. Decorate with fluting if you like. Wine glasses, wind players? Whatever works.

3. Cut a small vent to let steam escape.

4. Bake for 30 minutes until golden brown.

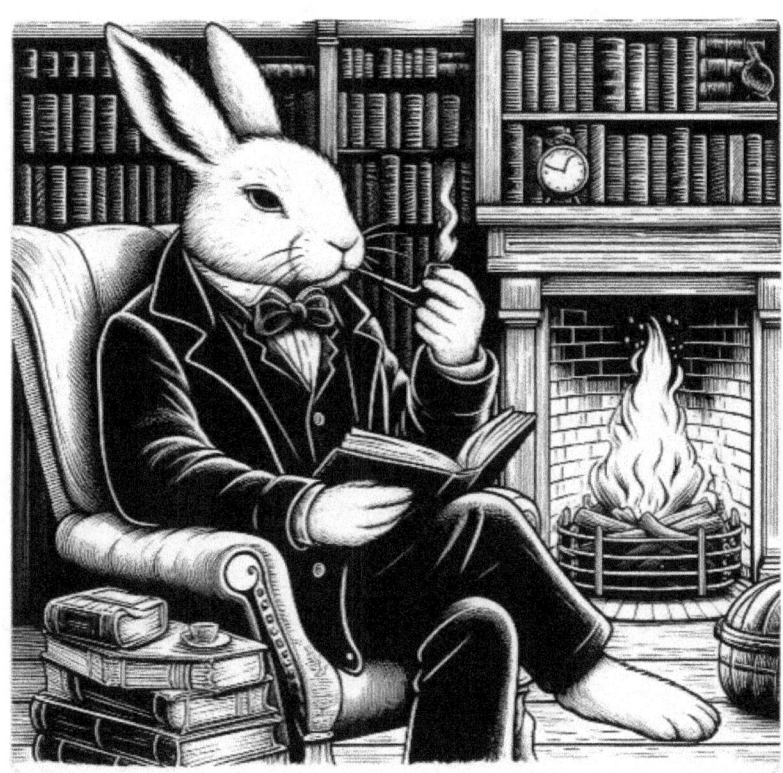

Rabbit Casserole

PREP overnight   COOK 1 to 2 hours   SERVES 6-8

INGREDIENTS

2 rabbits, jointed	1/2 lemon, juice only
6 tablespoons olive oil	2 ounces seasoned flour
4 garlic cloves, crushed	1 onion, sliced
1 sprig fresh rosemary	1 celery stalk, sliced
2 bay leaves	8 anchovy fillets in oil
1 pint dry white wine	3 ounces capers

DIRECTIONS

1. Preheat the oven to 325 F

2. Put rabbit pieces into a large bowl. Add three tablespoons of the olive oil, garlic, rosemary, bay leaves, white wine and lemon juice. Stir well, cover and marinate in the refrigerator overnight.

3. Remove the rabbit meat from the marinade, saving the marinade, and pat dry. Dust the rabbit pieces in the seasoned flour and shake off excess.

4. Heat the remaining olive oil in a large pan over a medium heat. Add the rabbit pieces to the hot oil and fry for 4-5 minutes, until golden-brown. Move the rabbit to an ovenproof casserole dish.

5. Pour the reserved marinade into the hot frying pan and warm through, then pour it into the casserole with the rabbit. Add the onion and celery to the casserole. Cook in the oven for 45 minutes, or until the rabbit is tender.

6. Add the anchovies and capers and cook for another 15 minutes.

SAUSAGE, MEATBALLS, MEATLOAF

Making Rabbit Sausage

This isn't so much a recipe as some general directions for the sausage-making process.

PREPARATION

1. Put deboned rabbit meat in the freezer for about 30 minutes to make it firm for grinding. Without this step, it can become soft or mushy during grinding.

2. Choose a medium grind with a plate hole size of 4-5 mm.

3. Put the rabbit meat through the grinder once, letting it go into a chilled bowl.

4. Add your seasonings and spices to the ground meat.

STUFFING THE CASINGS

Unless you have your own sheep or cows, you'll have to buy casings. There are several types and several kinds within each group:

1. **Collagen**

    ◆ Smoke Casing

    - Stronger than many other casings
    - Good for wieners, hot dogs, snack sticks
    - Inexpensive
    - Doesn't need to be soaked before use
    - Often peeled off before eating the sausage

    ◆ Fresh Casing

    - A soft casing
    - Good for tender meats that aren't going to be hung up
    - Good for breakfast sausage and bratwurst
    - Often peeled off before eating the sausage

2. **Natural** – natural casings have more 'snap' to them than collagen casings. They're preserved in saline or salt and so require some rinsing and soaking before making your sausage. They're

more expensive but also more flexible, tender, and durable. They're generally easier to handle, versatile for many sorts of sausages and have a texture that 'snaps' when you bite into the sausage. They make for a higher quality and better-tasting sausage than most casings.

- Sheep
  - Used on the most tender sausages
  - They're very small, which can limit their use
  - Can be used for hot dogs, snack sticks, breakfast sausage
- Beef
  - Beef bung caps
    - Good for large sausages
    - Can be used for mortadella, large bologna and souse sausages
  - Beef middles
    - This is a heavier casing
    - Removed rather than eaten
    - A good choice for for salami
  - Beef rounds
    - Very low fat
    - Very salty
    - These need to be rinsed, soaked in cold water ideally for several hours, then soaked in warm water, before use.
    - Good for blood sausage, ring bologna, and mettwurst
- Hog — a popular choice for rabbit sausage
  - Often used for traditional sausages, including kielbasa, bratwurst, and smoked Polish sausage

3. **Cellulose** – cellulose casings are made from the Abaca tree, so they can be used to make vegetarian sausage
   - Good for smoked sausage, pepperoni, bologna, summer sausage and others

- They should be soaked in warm water for half an hour before being used
- Because they're very stretchy, they can make very large sausages
- They're usually removed after cooking the sausage and before eating it

4. **Fibrous** — fibrous casings are made from cellulose and paper fibers
    - This is a particularly strong case, good for use with a sausage-stuffing machine
    - Soak before use
    - Good for large sausages

Soak the casings in warm water and rinse them thoroughly.

Feed the casings onto your sausage stuffer tube and tie a knot.

Guide the sausage mix into the stuffer.

Rabbit-Apple Sausage

PREP overnight + 15 minutes   COOK 10 minutes   SERVES 5-6

INGREDIENTS

6 pounds rabbit meat, cut up	3/4 teaspoon ground nutmeg
2 teaspoons salt	1/2 teaspoon ground cinnamon
1-1/2 teaspoons rubbed sage	1 cup finely chopped peeled tart apple
1-1/4 teaspoons white pepper	2 tablespoons canola oil

DIRECTIONS

1. Combine the first six ingredients in a bowl. The original recipe said in a large bowl. Recipes often specify bowl sizes. I trust you'll look at the ingredients and have a pretty good sense for the appropriate size and I don't need to specify. Whatever size bowl you use, cover the ingredients in it and refrigerate overnight.

2. The next day, mince that apple. Mince it good. [If you were born in the 80s or later, look up the reference. You may then dance, whipping your long hair around, while finishing this recipe. Trust me, it's more fun that way.]

3. Use a food processor to coarsely grind the refrigerated mixture into small batches. Stir in minced apple.

4. Shape into 16 patties, about 3 inches each. Heat oil in a skillet; cook patties over medium heat for 5 minutes on each side, until sausage is browned and meat is no longer pink.

Rabbit Sausage with Fennel, Chili Flakes and Broccoli Rabe

INGREDIENTS

3/4 cup kosher salt	9 pounds rabbit meat, shoulders, legs, loin, diced
3 tablespoons freshly ground black pepper	2-1/4 pound pork backfat, diced
3 tablespoons fennel seed	7 ounces buttermilk powder
2-1/2 tablespoons crushed red pepper	1 pound blanched broccoli rabe, chopped*
2 tablespoons sugar	2 cups ice-cold water
1-1/2 teaspoons finely chopped rosemary	Pork casing (approximately 20 feet in length)
1-1/2 teaspoons chopped fresh fennel fronds	

* Not to be confused with broccoli. Broccoli rabe (pronounced rahb) is a slightly bitter leafy green

DIRECTIONS

1. In a small bowl mix together salt, pepper, fennel seed, red pepper, sugar, rosemary, and fennel fronds to make your seasoning.

2. In a large bowl, season the rabbit meat and fat *lightly* with the seasoning, saving the rest for later.

3. Put the meat in the freezer. When frozen solid, break the mixture apart. Mix with the buttermilk powder and broccoli rabe.

4. Use a meat grinder to grind the mixture on the large die into a chilled bowl. Consider setting the chilled bowl in another bowl full of ice. Freeze the ground meat at least 20 minutes, then grind again through the small die. Put the meat in the bowl of a stand mixer fitted with the paddle attachment and beat it (just beat it!), slowly adding the ice water until fully mixed in.

5. Dampen the pork casing in cold water and fit the open end over the sausage stuffing tube. Bunch the entire casing over the tube. With the motor on slow, guide the meat into the casing until it is fully stuffed. The original recipe specifies to guide it *carefully*. I guess that's better than guiding it recklessly. So maybe don't have too many beers before this step. Be careful not to pack it too tightly by guiding the casing out along with the meat. Twist sections of the casing about 3 inches apart to form links of about 4 ounces each.

Parmesan Rabbit Sausage

INGREDIENTS

2 pounds ground rabbit	3 tablespoons fresh parsley
1 pound pork butt or pork shoulder, ground	1 tablespoon garlic
2-1/2 teaspoons salt	1 cup green onion or shallot
1/2 teaspoon black pepper	1/2 cup onion, minced
1/2 teaspoon ground cayenne pepper	1 egg
1/4 teaspoon white pepper	3/4 cup chicken stock or rabbit stock
1/2 teaspoon ground cumin	1/2 cup fine breadcrumbs
2 teaspoons fresh thyme, minced	2 tablespoons grated Parmesan cheese
1 tablespoon fresh oregano, minced	7 natural pork casings
1 tablespoon fresh basil minced	

DIRECTIONS

1. Peel and mince the garlic. Slice the green onions/shallot in thin slices. Mince the parsley.
2. Soak the casings in cool water for about five minutes to remove surface salt. Longer than 5 minutes will leave them too tender to stuff. Flush salt from the inside with cold water.
3. Gently squeeze water out; cover the rinsed casings and refrigerate them.
4. Combine all other ingredients in a large bowl; knead together thoroughly.
5. Put the sausage mix in a plastic container, cover and refrigerate for 24 hours.
6. Fill the casings, making links by twisting the sausage about every four inches for a regular serving, and less for appetizer sausages.
7. Preheat oven to 300°F.
8. Put the sausage links in a shallow pan with an inch of water; bake uncovered for an hour.
9. Place sausage links under broiler and cook until brown on top, about 5 minutes.
10. Serve hot.

Rabbit Sausage with Garlic and Sweet White Wine

INGREDIENTS

10 pounds rabbit meat in fist-sized chunks, frozen	4 teaspoons oregano
3-1/2 pounds of fatty pork shoulder, frozen	Citrus zest
1/3 cup of kosher salt	A bit of fennel seed
1/3 cup of black pepper	1 cup of sweet white wine
10-15 cloves of garlic, to taste	

DIRECTIONS

1. Put rabbit and pork through grinder together or one after another. Run it through again. So technically...run rabbit, run.

2. To get the last of the meat out of the grinder, run a piece or two of bread through the grinder. Stop as soon as you see the bread crumbs come out. Put the meat in the freezer while you clean the grinder.

3. Mix salt, oregano, pepper, garlic, fennel seed and most of the wine together in a bowl.

4. Take the meat from the freezer. Spoon about half the spiced wine onto the meat and fold it into the meat.

5. Add the rest and fold it into the meat.

6. Add the last of the wine to the meat and knead it all again, mixing well.

7. Stuff into 32-35 mm natural hog casings, using a sausage stuffing machine

Rabbit Meatloaf with Pepper Jack Cheese

INGREDIENTS

2 pounds ground rabbit	Olive oil
2 eggs	1 chopped onion
Cornmeal	Salt
Panko	Pepper
Barbecue sauce	Onion soup mix
Pepper jack cheese	Granulated garlic

DIRECTIONS

1. Preheat the oven to 375 F.
2. Put half the ground rabbit in an oiled loaf pan, add a layer of pepper jack cheese and cover it lightly with the remaining meat.
3. Sprinkle the top with cornmeal, panko, and Parmesan cheese.
4. Bake for 45 min.

Rabbit Meatballs

PREP 10 minutes   COOK 20 minutes   SERVES 3-4

INGREDIENTS

1 pound ground rabbit meat	1 egg
1/2 cup of Italian-style bread crumbs	Pi Pizza spice blend
1/2 cup of Parmesan cheese	

DIRECTIONS

1. Preheat oven to 400 F.
2. Mix all the ingredients together.
3. Shape into balls of about an inch in diameter and place on parchment sheet or on a greased pan.
4. Bake for 20 minutes.

The recipe given here was originally for beef meatballs. It's open to numerous substitutions. The bread crumbs can be any bread crumbs. Other types of cheese can be substituted for the Parmesan.

Rabbit meat is more delicate and might be served well by adding finely minced shallots and seasoning it with sage, savory, and a sweeter spice such as nutmeg.

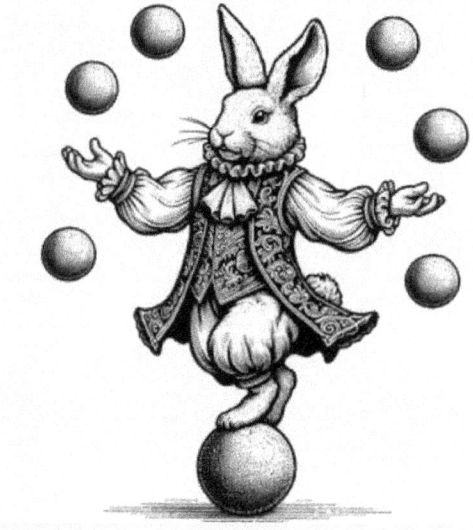

MUFFINS, MISCELLANEOUS

Muffins with Rabbit Meat and Cheese

I think muffins made with rabbit meat qualifies for the Things I Never Thought I'd See category! It also seems like a good paraphrase for the old poem, *I never saw a purple cow….I never want to see one!* However, I'm 'game' to try a rabbit meat muffin!

INGREDIENTS

2 cups flour	2 eggs
5-1/3 ounces rabbit fillet	4 tablespoons olive oil
2 teaspoons baking powder	1/2 teaspoon salt
8-1/2 ounces natural yogurt	1/2 teaspoon baking soda
3/4 cup mozzarella	

DIRECTIONS

1. Preheat oven to 355 F.
2. Boil the rabbit fillet until cooked and cut into small cubes.
3. Cut the mozzarella into cubes.
4. Mix flour with baking powder, soda and salt.
5. In another bowl, beat eggs with yogurt and olive oil.
6. Mix flour into yogurt and eggs. Add the meat and cheese and mix again. (I guess that's a remix?)
7. Put the finished dough into molds, fill them 2/3 and bake for 30 minutes.
8. Cool the prepared cupcakes a little, then remove from the mold and serve.

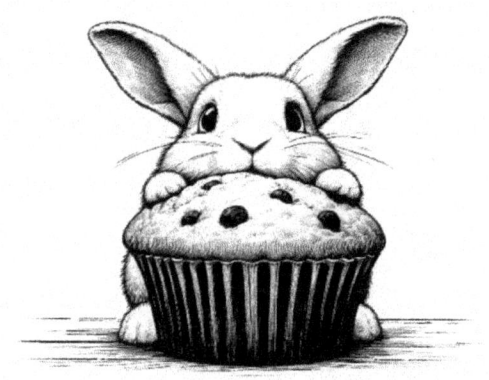

Rabbit and Gorgonzola Tart

PREP: 25 MINUTES   COOK: 50 MINUTES   SERVES 6

INGREDIENTS

1 ready-made short crust pastry	1 egg
14 ounces rabbit fillet	1 cup liquid cream
1 onion	2 tablespoons capers
6 leaves basil	1 tablespoon honey
7 ounces crumbled gorgonzola	1 tablespoon olive oil
1-1/2 ounces butter	Salt and freshly ground pepper

DIRECTIONS

1. Preheat the oven at 350° F
2. Butter a rectangular tart mold. Roll out the short crust dough. Prick the base with a fork.
3. Cut the rabbit fillets into cubes. Peel and chop the onions. Heat the oil and the rest of the butter in a pan. Stir the rabbit and onions in the pan for 5 minutes with a wooden spoon.
4. Add the honey, salt and pepper. Cook 3 more minutes, stirring constantly.
5. Rinse, dry and chop the basil.
6. Break the egg in a bowl and beat together with the cream. Mix in the capers and crumbled Gorgonzola. Add the basil. Salt lightly and add pepper to taste.
7. Lay out the rabbit cubes across the dough. Cover with Gorgonzola.
8. Bake 40 minutes. Serve with green salad and freshly steamed spinach seasoned with salt, pepper and drizzled with olive oil.

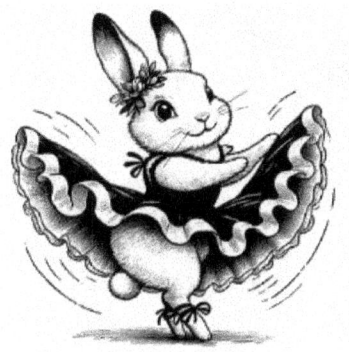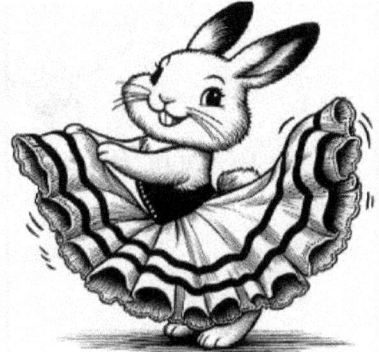

Orange Rabbit with Thermomix

INGREDIENTS

2 pounds of rabbit in pieces	1 teaspoon dried thyme
Juice of two oranges	1/4 cup soy sauce
5-1/2 ounces white wine	3-1/2 tablespoons honey
5 cloves of garlic	Salt
2-2/3 ounces olive oil	Orange slices to decorate

DIRECTIONS

1. Cut the rabbit into pieces, sprinkle a little salt and set aside for a few minutes.
2. Put the garlic cloves in the Thermomix bowl, and program for 5 seconds / Speed 5. With the help of a spatula or spoon, lower the garlic remains adhering to the walls and lid of the Thermomix bowl to the blades. Pour in the oil, program 5 minutes / 120 ° C / Speed 1.
3. Add the rabbit, thyme, soy sauce, honey and orange juice to the Thermomix bowl, program 15 minutes / 120 ° C / Reverse rotation / Bucket speed.
4. Pour it onto a serving dish. This meal goes well with any grilled vegetable.

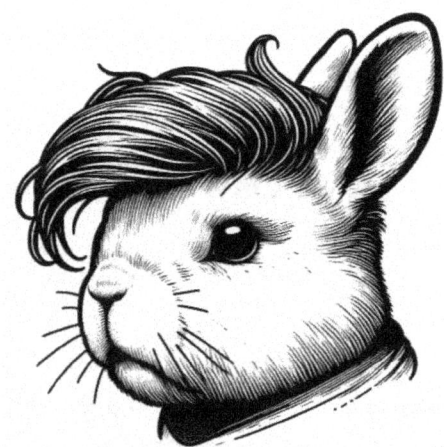

Orange Rabbit Good!

Sous Vide

Sous vide is a cooking method developed in the 1970s. It involves putting food in a heat-proof bag or glass jar which is then immersed in hot water. This recipe calls for a sous vide machine which will likely cost you well over $300. You can, however, use this technique with a pot of water, Ziploc bags, a binder clip, and an accurate thermometer. The technique is as follows:

1. Fill a pot with as much water as it can hold without overflowing once you add your food.

2. Ideally, secure your thermometer inside the pot with a heavy-duty binder clip so you can constantly monitor the temperature. Attach the clip to the side with the 'pinchers' flipped up. Slide the thermometer through both of them so the tip is inside the liquid but not touching the bottom of the pot.

3. Bring the water to the correct temperature. You may have to adjust the heat or move the pot around the stove to keep it within a degree or two of the necessary temperature.

4. Put the food to be cooked into the Ziploc bags. *Do not overfill!* To seal, keep the open end up while pushing down in water *without letting water in the top.* Then seal the bag.

5. Submerge the bags of food in the heated water. Clipping the bags to the side with more binder clips can help keep them submerged and make it easier to get them out.

6. The temperature will drop when you add the food. Raise the heat gradually to bring it back up.

For the following recipe, I'll be giving the directions that don't require the machine.

Fried Rabbit Sous Vide

PREP 1-1/2 – 12 hours	COOK 45-60 minutes	SERVES 8-9

INGREDIENTS

Brine	*Batter*
2-1/2 cups water	Reserved cooking liquid from rabbit
2 tablespoons kosher salt, fine grind	1-1/2 teaspoons kosher salt
1-1/2 to 2 teaspoons hot pepper sauce	1-1/2 teaspoons hot pepper sauce, or to taste
2-1/2 tablespoons brown sugar	Juice of 1 medium lemon, freshly squeezed
12-1/2 pounds whole rabbit, in 6-8 pieces	1/4 cup masa harina/corn flour
4 whole bay leaves	1/4 cup flour
	As needed peanut oil

DIRECTIONS

Preheat the sous vide machine or your water to 139°F/59°C.

Brine

1. In a large bowl mix the salt, sugar, hot sauce and water stirring constantly until the salt and sugar are completely dissolved.
2. Marinate the rabbit in this sauce overnight in the refrigerator. (A sous vide machine has a function that will do it in less than two hours.)
3. Remove the rabbit from the marinade and seal it in bags with the bay leaves.
4. Cook in the pre-heated water for 45 minutes to 1 hour.

Batter

1. Remove the rabbit from the bags and save the cooking liquid which should be about 1/2 a cup.
2. Heat the peanut oil over medium-high heat until the oil reaches 375°F on a deep-frying/candy thermometer.
3. Line a baking sheet with paper towels or a wire cooling rack.
4. Add salt, hot pepper sauce and lemon juice to the saved rabbit cooking liquid. Blend well.
5. In a large bowl combine the masa harina corn flour and flour and using the flavored cooking liquid to make a thin batter. If there is not sufficient liquid for the batter add poultry broth or water to reach the desired consistency.
6. Add the cooked rabbit to the bowl, coating each piece with a thin layer of batter.
7. Keeping the temperature at 375°F, fry the rabbit in the oil until the batter is crispy and golden, about 3-5 minutes. Put fried rabbit on the baking sheet to drain, about 3 minutes.
8. Repeat: Working in batches, using the remaining rabbit.
9. Serve with your favorite sides.

In Northern Europe there was a belief that witches might take the form of hares in order to cause mischief, such as stealing milk from cows. Naturally, others wanted to scare away these mischief-makers which may have given rise to the custom of the Hare Pie Scramble in Hallaton, Leicestershire, England, in which villagers scrambled to eat a piece of hare pie.

I guess fear of being turned into a hare pie would scare me!

A parson in 1790 tried to stop the tradition but it continues to this day—or at least up to the day the blog entry was made that reports this story.

Rabbit Organ Meat Saute with Garlic Cream Bone Broth Sauce

INGREDIENTS

Organ Meat	*Reduction Sauce*
Organ meat from 4-6 rabbits	1/2 cup bone broth
Bacon fat or butter	1/3 cup heavy cream
Sea salt	1/4 cup butter
Freshly ground pepper	3 cloves garlic crushed or minced
	1/8 teaspoon sea salt

DIRECTIONS

1. Saute the organ meat in bacon fat or butter with salt and pepper.
2. Set the sauteed organs in a warm oven or on pre-warmed plates while you make the reduction cream sauce.
3. Crush or mince the garlic. Add it, with butter and salt, to the pan in which the organs were sauteed, over low heat.
4. About 30 seconds after garlic begins to sizzle add the broth.
5. De-glaze the pan. Scrape up any remaining bits of organ meat with a spatula.
6. Turn the heat to medium until the broth comes to a boil; turn it down to low and let the garlic simmer for 3-5 minutes.
7. Add the heavy cream and reduce the sauce for another 2-3 minutes.
8. Serve on warmed plates with the reduction sauce spooned over the meat. Great sides are cheese, salad greens, roast rabbit or chicken, and vegetables. A strong, richly-flavored wine such as a glass of Cabernet Sauvignon.

VARIOUS COUNTRIES

Not surprisingly, rabbit has been cooked in virtually every country, throughout time. Enjoy a few recipes from around the world.

Rabbit Curry—Indian

This can be made with jackrabbit which is a dark meat, or with rabbit, which is a white meat. Really it can be made with any meat. But this is a rabbit cookbook. So use rabbit.

PREP 15 minutes	COOK 45 minutes	SERVES 4

INGREDIENTS

1/4 cup ghee, clarified butter, or vegetable oil	2 cups water
2 pounds hare or rabbit meat, cut into chunks	2 bay leaves
Salt	1 heaping teaspoon turmeric
2 cups yellow or white onion, sliced root to tip	1/4 cup Madras curry paste, or 2
2 tablespoons minced ginger	tablespoons Madras curry powder
A 14-ounce can of tomato puree	1 tablespoon Garam Masala
1 cup plain yogurt, Greek style is best	1/4 cup chopped cilantro for garnish

DIRECTIONS

1. Heat the clarified butter in a wide pot, either a sauce pot or high-sided frying pan, over medium-high heat. Pat the rabbit pieces dry with paper towels and brown them well. Salt the meat as it cooks. When it's browned, move it to a bowl.

2. Add the onion and sauté until it begins to brown at the edges, about 5 minutes. Add the ginger and garlic and cook another minute.

3. Return the rabbit to the pot and add the tomato puree, water, bay leaves, turmeric and Madras curry paste. Stir in the yogurt and bring to a low simmer. Salt to taste and simmer 30 minutes.

4. Stir in the Garam Masala and cilantro.

5. Serve on rice with a hoppy beer

Rabbit in Mustard Sauce — French

Rabbit in mustard sauce—lapin à la moutarde—is a French bistro classic. Braising the rabbit in the rich mustard sauce gives especially succulent, tender meat. Soak up the sauce with crusty bread.

INGREDIENTS

1 3- to 4-lb rabbit, cut into 6-8 pieces	2-1/2 cups chicken stock or broth
Salt and pepper	2 tablespoons whole-grain mustard
1-1/2 tablespoons butter	3-4 sprigs of thyme
1-1/2 tablespoons oil	12 sage leaves
1 medium onion or 4 shallots, diced	1/2 cup crème fraiche
2 tablespoons flour	2 teaspoons chopped capers
1 cup dry white wine	Sliced chives for garnish

DIRECTIONS

1. Season the rabbit with salt and pepper.
2. Heat a Dutch oven or large, deep, heavy pan over medium-high heat. Add butter and oil. When sizzling, sear the rabbit in batches, 3 to 4 minutes per side, until browned. Remove from pan and set aside.
3. Add the onion/shallot and sauté 5-6 minutes until soft and light brown, stirring occasionally.
4. Sprinkle onions with flour and stir until well mixed, then cook for a minute or so. Add wine and 1 cup broth, whisking as the sauce thickens. Whisk in remaining broth and 1 tablespoon of mustard and bring to a simmer. Taste for salt and adjust.
5. Return browned rabbit to the sauce. Add thyme and sage. Cover and simmer until meat is fork tender, 45 to 50 minutes.
6. Remove rabbit pieces from sauce, set aside, and keep warm. Put saucepan over medium heat and bring contents to a simmer. Whisk in crème fraîche, 1 tablespoon of mustard, and capers and simmer until somewhat thickened, about 5 minutes. Taste sauce and adjust seasoning.
7. Move rabbit to a warmed serving bowl and ladle the sauce over. Sprinkle with chives.

Civet of Hare or Jugged Hare—French

This recipe is known in Britain as Jugged Hare. In France it's called *Civet de Lievre*. It's a recipe our Founding Fathers would have eaten but it goes back even before Jamestown.

Hares, or jackrabbits, have tougher meat than rabbits. They have red meat like beef, not white, like rabbits or chickens. Jugged, which can be done with many animals, means the sauce is thickened with the blood and liver of the animal, and pureed with heavy cream. In place of a hare liver, you can use duck or chicken liver. Puree it in a blender with the heavy cream, then stir this mixture into your finished sauce to thicken it.

Jugged hare takes time and must be done precisely but you'll love it!

PREP 1-2 days plus 15 minutes   COOK 3 hours   SERVES 8

INGREDIENTS

1 hare or 3 cottontail rabbits, or 2 domestic rabbits	1/4 pound bacon
Blood from the hare mixed with a little red wine vinegar (optional)	5 tablespoons duck fat or butter
	1/2 ounce dried mushrooms (chanterelles are good)
2 carrots, grated	
2 celery sticks, minced	1 tablespoon sugar
1 large onion, grated	1 teaspoon quatre spices
3 bay leaves	1 pint stock or broth (any kind)
1 tablespoon dried thyme	1/4 pound fresh mushrooms
1 tablespoon chopped fresh rosemary	1 onion, sliced
1/4 cup brandy	1 tablespoon heavy cream
1 bottle red wine	1 tablespoon minced parsley
Flour for dusting	Salt and black pepper

DIRECTIONS

Marinade
1. Pour the brandy and wine into a pot. Bring to a boil for a few minutes to burn off most of the alcohol, then turn off the heat.

2. Cut the hare into large pieces: back legs, front legs, saddle into several sections — feel between vertebrae for places to chop with a cleaver or heavy knife. Salt it lightly.

3. While the wine-brandy broth is warm, pour it into a bowl or plastic bin big enough for the rabbits. Add onion, carrot, celery, rosemary, bay leaves, and thyme. Mix well.

4. When the wine mixture is room temperature, add the hare pieces. Cover and marinate in the refrigerator for 1-2 days.

Stew

1. Take the hare out of the marinade and pat it dry.

2. Strain the marinade through a fine-meshed sieve into a bowl. Set aside the vegetables.

3. Pour the marinade into a pot and bring to a boil. A layer of scum will form on top. Skim it off. Bring the marinade to a simmer. Skim the liquid a few times until it is clear, then turn off the heat.

4. Heat half the fat or lard in a large pot over medium-high heat.

5. Dust the pieces of hare in flour. While you can use white flour, using rye or another type of flour adds a unique flavor to the stew. Brown the rabbit meat in the pot in batches. When browned, set aside.

6. Heat another tablespoon or two of the fat or lard in a large frying pan over medium-high heat. When it's hot, turn the heat down to medium-low and add the pancetta. If you're using bacon, only use enough goose fat to lubricate the bottom of the pan, as the bacon should be fatty enough.

7. Preheat the oven to 300 degrees.

8. Cook the pancetta or bacon until crispy. Remove and set aside.

9. Add the vegetables to the frying pan you cooked the pancetta in, and turn the heat all the way up. It will sputter. (Let's hope it doesn't fume and rage!) Stir the vegetables, adding fat or lard as needed. Once they are coated and much of the liquid has steamed off, turn the heat down to medium and cook until they caramelize, about 10-12 minutes. Stir occasionally.

10. Return the hare to the Dutch oven and add the pancetta or bacon. Pour over the wine-brandy broth, then add the vegetables. Add the dried chanterelles, quatre pices and the sugar. Make sure everything is evenly distributed.

11. If you think you need more liquid, add stock. Bring it to a simmer and salt to taste.

12. Cover and put in the oven for 2-1/2 to 3 hours for a hare, 90 minutes for rabbits.

MAKING A STEW A CIVET

1. When the hare is almost falling off the bone, remove it from the pot. Set aside to cool.

2. While the meat is cooling, run everything left in the pot through a food mill with a medium plate. If you don't have a food mill, run it through a food processor or immersion blender. If you are doing this you really should push the blended mix through a sieve or chinois to catch any lumpy bits.

3. Clean the Dutch oven, or get another large, lidded pot.

4. Pick the meat from the bones of the hare. Try to keep the meat in large pieces and be careful to get rid of all small bones.

5. Return the strained, blended stew to the pot, and add the chile paste, the onion previously sliced into half-moons, and the fresh chanterelles. Bring to a simmer, cover and cook for 20 minutes, or until the onions are nice and soft.

6. Return the pieces of hare to the pot and retest for salt. Add generous amounts of black pepper.

7. Blend the liver, blood and heavy cream together in a blender.

8. When the hare is warm, turn off the heat. Wait until all bubbles have simmered down, then add a ladelful of the stew to the mix of blood, liver, and heavy cream. Stir well. Repeat. Pour the mixture into the pot and stir it in to combine. Let it thicken. DO NOT LET THIS BOIL. You can still eat it if it does. It just won't look as good.

9. Top with parsley and serve with crusty bread, a green salad, and red wine.

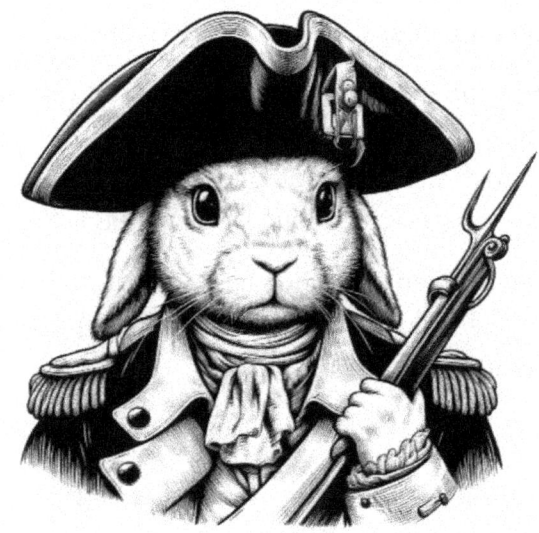

Sichuan Rabbit with Peanuts — Chinese

INGREDIENTS

Rabbit	Scallions
Chile paste	Peanuts, toasted and ground
Black bean paste	Sichuan peppercorns, toasted and ground
Soy	Toasted sesame seeds, toasted and ground

DIRECTIONS

1. Braise the rabbit, then pull the meat off the bones. Cut the meat into cubes; toss them with chili paste, black bean paste, soy, scallions and peanuts.

2. Consider adding Sichuan peppercorns and toasted sesame seeds, toasted and ground. Sichuan peppercorns can be found in some supermarkets, or bought online. There isn't a substitute for them. They're optional. The meal will still taste good, but they're part of what makes the flavors authentic.

The Chinese have a myth of the Jade Rabbit (who is actually white) who lives on the moon in a palace. The story starts when three sages, disguised as poor old hungry men, meet a rabbit who has nothing to give them. So he jumps into the fire, sacrificing himself to feed them. As a reward, he is granted immortality to live in a jade palace on the moon, where he can be seen making the Elixir of Life by pounding medicinal herbs with a pestle and mortar. He symbolizes self-sacrifice, kindness, compassion, and piety.

Spicy Cold Rabbit Meat – Chinese

The flavor of this dish is known as Zigong,

PREP 15 minutes   COOK 25 minutes   SERVES 2

INGREDIENTS

10 ounces rabbit meat	Light soy sauce
Salt	Bell peppers
Garlic	Blend oil
Chinese prickly ash	Cooking wine
Ginger	

DIRECTIONS

1. Wash rabbit meat and cut it into small pieces.   Chop the ginger.
2. Add the ginger, garlic and salt to the meat. Add light soy sauce and cooking wine. Mix well. Set aside for twenty minutes.
3. Slice and dice the Sichuan peppercorns and set aside.
4. Heat a large wok-style frying pan and put plenty of oil on the bottom. Bring the oil's temperature to about 70 degrees and turn to medium heat. Then put the rabbit meat into the pot.
5. Stir-fry until the pan is almost dry and turn the heat down to low. Add chili and peppercorns. Stir fry well, about 5 minutes.
6. Let cool to make spicy *cold* rabbit meat.

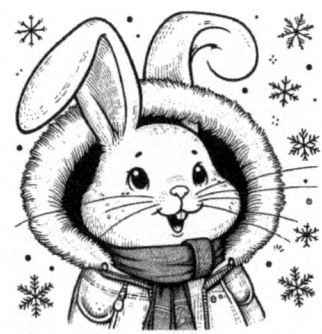

Cooking with Rabbit

Sweet and Sour Rabbit – Asian style

INGREDIENTS

1 whole rabbit, 3 pounds	1/3 cup pine nuts
Olive oil	1/3 cup blanched almonds
1 red onion	1/2 teaspoon ground cloves
5 ripe cherry tomatoes	2/3 cup full-bodied Sicilian red wine
1 fresh red chili	1/2 cup thick balsamic vinegar
5 fresh bay leaves	1 tablespoon runny honey

DIRECTIONS

1. Skin and joint the rabbit, keeping the offal (it's good stuff). Put it all in a cold casserole pan with 3 tablespoons of oil. Cook on medium-high, turning the rabbit occasionally, till it's golden-brown.

2. Mince the onion, quarter the tomatoes, cut the chili in half and remove the seeds. Add chilis, onions, bay, nuts, cloves and wine to the pan. Add 1-1/2 cups of water, bring to the boil, then simmer on low for 15 minutes.

3. Add balsamic and honey. Cook, stirring occasionally, until the rabbit is soft and tender and the liquid has reduced to a dark, thick coating—about 30 minutes. Serve hot or at room temperature. Serve with rice, pasta, bread or a salad.

Rabbit Ragu with Prosciutto—Italian

PREP 30-40 minutes   COOKS 4 hours 50 minutes   SERVES 6

INGREDIENTS

1-1/4 ounces pancetta	3 ounces white wine
2 stalks of celery	1 fresh red chili pepper
1 small leek	17 ounces organic vegetable stock
1 carrot	18 ounces tagliolini
1 onion	4 tablespoons mascarpone cheese
2 cloves of garlic	1 lemon
1/2 a bunch of fresh parsley	1-1/2 tablespoons butter
1 ounce pork fat	1/2 cup Parmesan cheese
1-1/4 ounces prosciutto fat	Pangratto*
1 cup wild rabbit meat, deboned and diced	Olive oil
1 fresh bay leaf	1 clove of garlic
1/2 a small bunch of fresh sage	1/2 cup breadcrumbs
2 sprigs of fresh rosemary	

* Crispy, flavorful Italian bread crumbs. If you can't find any, feel free to use any breadcrumbs.

DIRECTIONS

Ragù

1. Preheat the oven to 250° F
2. Dice pancetta. Trim, peel, and mince the celery, leek, carrot, onion, garlic, and parsley leaves.
3. Chop and melt the fats in a casserole pan on low heat. Add rabbit and pancetta and cook on medium until golden, about 5 to 8 minutes.
4. Add the vegetables, garlic, parsley and bay and cook until soft, about 5 minutes.
5. Chop the sage and rosemary leaves; add them, with wine, to the pan. Simmer for 5 minutes, or until the wine is reduced by half.
6. Chop the chili pepper; stir it in with the stock, and season.
7. Cook, covered, in the oven for 3 to 4 hours.

Pasta and Putting it Together

1. As the cooking time is nearly done, boil the pasta, drain, and rinse.

2. Bring the ragù to a boil on the stove; remove from the heat and keep warm.

3. Heat 2 tablespoons of oil in a pan. Peel and smash the garlic, and fry it in the pan until golden. Add the breadcrumbs and season. Fry on high, tossing regularly, until golden and crunchy.

4. Drain and add the pasta to the ragù along with the mascarpone, lemon juice and butter, and season. Stir well and let sit for 1 minute to allow the pasta to absorb the sauce.

5. Serve with grated Parmesan, pangrattato and lemon zest.

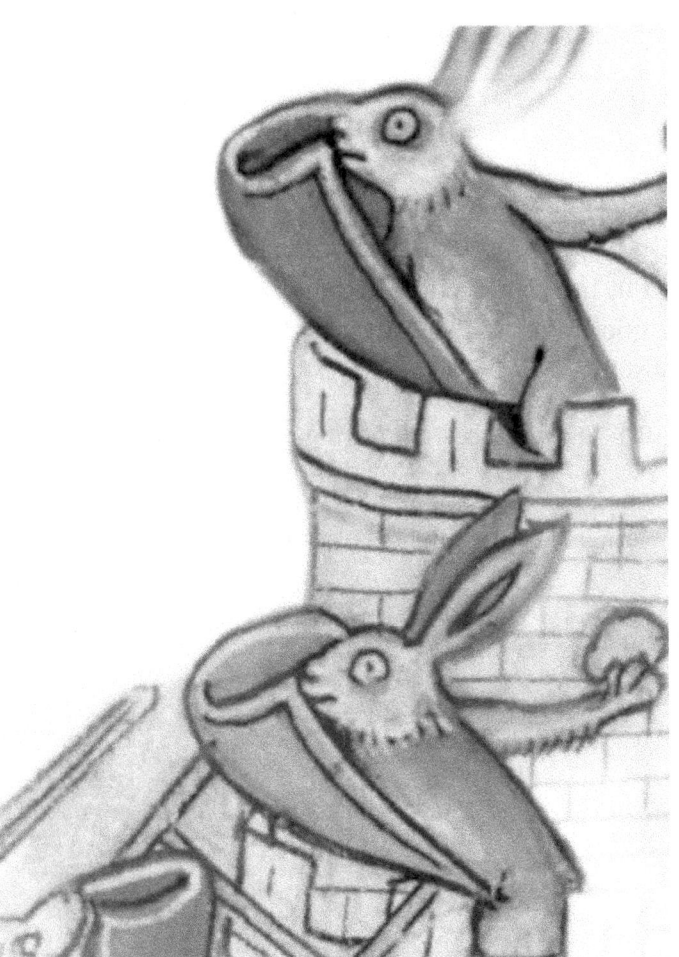

Was Monty Python completely wrong in their depiction of the killer rabbit?

In a strange contrast to the rabbit symbolizing fertility, life, and rebirth, medieval art often depicted rabbits as violent. The theory is that their ability to reproduce and spread is analogous to the way evil spreads and harms the world. By that analogy, the rabbit was a symbol of evil. It's interesting that this resonates with African and Indian cultures, who saw rabbits as wily tricksters.

The story of the tortoise and the hare, for example, shows the rabbit as cunning and proud. In both ancient Greek mythology and African Bushmen folklore, rabbits are scheming villains.

Similarly, in the Middle Ages, the rabbit was a symbol of evil, reflected here in just one example

Calabrian Rabbit with Red Peppers

Calabrian food is of the region in southern Italy

PREP 20 minutes   COOK 1 hour 15 minute   SERVES 4

INGREDIENTS

1 store-bought rabbit or 2 cottontails	2 tablespoons dried oregano or marjoram
3 tablespoons olive oil	1/2 cup crushed tomatoes
Salt	1 tablespoon Calabrian hot pepper paste
3 bay leaves	OR 2 teaspoons Sriracha hot sauce
1/2 pound Italian sausage	2 tablespoons sweet paprika
4 garlic cloves, smashed	1 cup roasted red peppers, cut into slices

DIRECTIONS

1. Cut the Italian sausage into large pieces.
2. Cut the rabbits into serving-sized pieces. Put them in a wide, shallow pot, just barely covered with water. Bring to a simmer and add a good pinch of salt and the bay leaves. Skim off any scum that forms on the surface of the water.
3. Simmer the rabbit uncovered for 1 hour, turning the pieces from time to time as the water cooks away; this keeps both sides moist.
4. Add the remaining ingredients and mix well. Keep turning the rabbit and sausage to be sure they're coated in the sauce.
5. Let the sauce thickens for 10-15 minutes and serve!

Belgian Rabbit Legs

INGREDIENTS

1/4 cup olive oil	2-1/2 cups Chicken stock
20 rabbit legs, skinless, bone in	1-3/4 cups Golden raisins
5-3/4 cups yellow onions, diced	1 teaspoon nutmeg, ground
12-3/4 cups white mushrooms, fresh, sliced	1 tablespoon sugar, fine, granulated
1-1/2 cups all-purpose flour	1 tablespoon Kosher salt
8 cups dark Belgian ale	2 teaspoons Black pepper
10 oz tomato paste, canned	

DIRECTIONS

1. Preheat oven to 325 F.
2. Heat olive oil in a large pan on medium high. Sauté rabbit legs in batches until golden brown all over. Move the meat to two large 2-inch deep pans.
3. Sauté onions and mushrooms on medium heat in the pan used to cook the rabbit. Cover the pan to sweat the vegetables for 5 minutes. Remove cover and sauté vegetables until tender.
4. Add flour and cook, stirring occasionally, until light brown in color, forming a roux, then stir in Belgian ale and tomato paste. Simmer, reduce heat to low and cook for about 20 minutes, until liquid is reduced by half. Stir in chicken stock, raisins, nutmeg, sugar, salt and pepper.
5. Pour the Belgian ale sauce over rabbit and cover the pans with foil.
6. Bake 2'10 to 2'30", turning rabbit legs over to evenly coat with sauce halfway through baking. When the rabbit is so tender it's falling off the bone, take the pans from oven and move rabbit to large platter. Keep warm.
7. Pour the sauce into a large saucepan. Cook over medium heat, stirring occasionally until the sauce is thick, about 30 minutes
8. Put a rabbit leg on each plate and drizzle it with Belgian ale sauce. Serve immediately.

Hungarian Rabbit Paprikash

INGREDIENTS

1-1/2 pounds boneless skinless rabbit meat	2-1/4 cups water
1-2 tablespoons oil	3/4 cup flour
4 tablespoons Hungarian paprika	
3 tablespoons onion powder	*Dumplings:*
2 teaspoons salt	6 eggs
1/4 teaspoon pepper	4 cups flour
32 ounces chicken broth	1-1/2 cups water
10 ounces sour cream	1/2 teaspoon salt

DIRECTIONS

1. Start water boiling for the dumplings. While it boils, remove fat from the chicken, tenderize it, and cut into bite-sized pieces. Brown rabbit in oil a large pan on medium-high heat for 6-10 minutes.

2. Stir paprika, onion powder, salt, pepper, and chicken broth in with the rabbit. Bring to a boil, lower heat, put on a lid and simmer for 25 minutes.

3. Stir water, flour and sour cream together in a bowl until smooth. Cover and set aside.

4. Mix eggs, flour, water, and salt for the dumplings together in a bowl to make a thick, dry mix. If it's too gooey, add small amounts of flour until it is more dry.

5. When the water boils, turn the heat to low. Rest the bowl on the edge of the pot, tipping it till the dumpling dough rests at the edge. Use a table knife to slice small chunks of dough into the pot. Repeat until all of the dough has been used. Dip the knife occasionally into the boiling water to prevent the dough sticking to it. Raise heat and boil dumplings about 5-6 minutes.

6. When the rabbit is almost done simmering, spoon some of its sauce into the sour cream/flour/water mix to keep the sour cream from curdling. Put the lid on and shake it up, baby, now shake it up good! Twist and shout! Be sure there are no chunks in the mix, then stir it into the rabbit pan. Mix until consistent. Stirring occasionally, bring the sauce to a boil for sauce to thicken.

7. Drain the water from the dumplings. Serve the rabbit and sauce on top of the dumplings.

The Hungarian Giant Rabbit is actually on the small side for a 'giant,' weighing in at 12 to 14 pounds. They come in a variety of colors and have a docile and inquisitive nature. It is now an endangered breed.

In times past, Hungarian folklore taught that they were spiritual guardians of home and family.

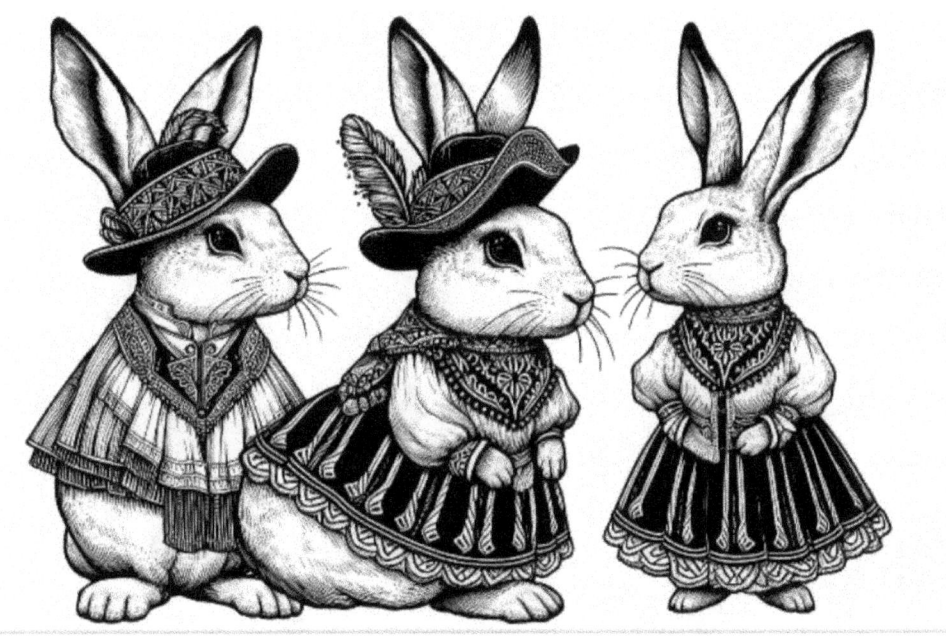

Rabbits do not wear clothes.

MEDIEVAL RECIPES

Reading a medieval cookbook is a different experience from reading a modern one. We view cooking as more of a science of mixing exact amounts in exact ways to exactly reproduce the same result. They're a bit like a science experiment in that respect. They're also written with the idea of people learning.

A medieval cookbook, by contrast, has less information. It tends to have the ingredients with either no amount specified or a generalized term in lieu of an exact amount. They were likely used primarily by those who had been cooking for years, using very different methods than we use today. In that time, any woman (we're going to assume it's a woman for the moment) of a class to be cooking (in other words not royalty) would likely have been working beside her mother from her earliest years, watching by observing and then by actively helping even as young as six or seven.

If she was cooking in a manor home or castle, she probably had an 'internship' and had done so much cooking that she didn't need exact measurements or temperatures. She probably knew her employer's taste and knew if he liked more or less spice, more or less of a certain vegetable, more or less meat.

Cooking was both a learned skill and an art. The experience of the cook and her use of a cookbook would be very different from the audience for cookbooks today. Sometimes we can find modern variations on these recipes. However, I'm going to leave them much as they were written.

There are relatively few cookbooks remaining from medieval times, so who knows what we'd learn if we had more still available to us. Use the recipes here as starting points.

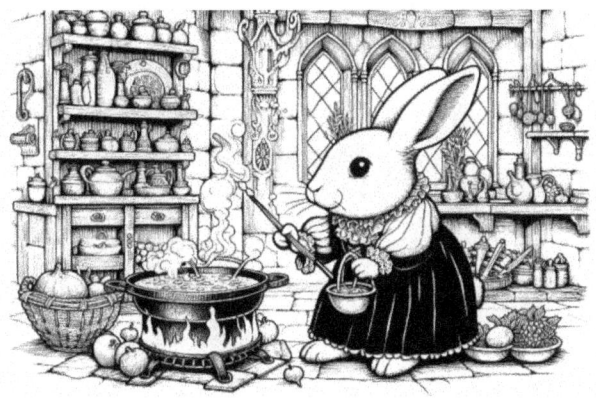

Rabbit—Then and Now

The modern American may have an image of rabbits being snared, shot, or hunted by fur traders in the seventeenth century, in colonial times or more recently by Appalachian farmers. It was 'free food,' and therefore might be seen as poor man's fare

By contrast, rabbit farming was a lucrative business in medieval times. Historian Paul Murphy writes, "a single rabbit in the thirteenth century was worth 3 1/2d. and another 1d. for its fur, far more than a craftsman's daily wage, maybe five times the price of a chicken and was the equivalent in price of a suckling pig."

Another English history site backs up this information that one rabbit cost more than a workman's daily wage. In today's terms, a workman might be anything from a 16-year-old at a fast-food place who might earn $80 for a day's work to a construction worker who would earn $200-$300 for a day's work. A rabbit, then, might cost the ordinary man between $80 and $300 for probably less than 10 pounds of meat. This is expensive indeed!

It's easy to see why rabbits were considered luxury food, but they also provided both clothing. Thus it was a status symbol to wear or eat rabbit. It was also a symbol of wealth to farm your own. Rabbits in that time had many predators (they still do). To raise them, keep them close for harvesting, and protect them from predators meant you had the land for a warren. Lords with the wealth and status to own deer parks might also keep warrens.

Monastic houses were particularly fond of raising rabbits. Apart from food and income, rabbit farming was likened to shepherding and rabbits were associated with the resurrection of Jesus.

Rabbit in Gravy—Coneys in Gravy

This recipe comes from the 1430 book *Liber Cure Cocorum,* "The Art of Cookery," which likely came from the Lancashire region. If you read the northern English dialect of the 15th century, you'll do well with the original.

INGREDIENTS

Rabbits	Cloves or Ginger
Almond Milk	Wine or Sugar
Grated Bread or Wheat Starch	Water

DIRECTIONS

Seethe well your coneys in clear water,

After, in cold water you wash them separately,

Take milk of almonds, mix it anon

With grated bread or amidon (wheat starch);

Season it with cloves or good ginger;

Boil it over the fire,

Hew the coneys, put them thereto,

Season it with wine or sugar then.

Coneys are rabbits.
You can buy almond milk, or soak almonds in water for 12 hours, drain the remaining water, blend it all and drain it through cheesecloth.

Rabbit in Wine Currant Sauce

This recipe comes from the 14th century English cookbook, *Forme of Cury*

ORIGINAL (good luck!)

Connynges in Cyrip:

Take connynges and seeþ hem wel in good broth. Take wyne greke and do þerto with a porcioun of vynegar and flour of canel, hoole clowes, quybibes hoole, and ooþer gode spices, with raisouns coraunce and gyngyuer ypared and ymynced. Take vp the connynges and smyte hem on pecys and cast hem in to the siryppe, and seeþ hem a litel in fere, and serue it forth.

INGREDIENTS	
Whole rabbit or pieces	Spices: 'Cinnamon, whole cloves, whole cubebs, and any other good spices' ***
Broth (of whatever sort you have)	
Greek wine *	Currants
Vinegar **	Fresh ginger root

*A sweet Italian wine is suggested.

**Red wine vinegar would be a good choice

***Other good spices could mean researching spices used in medieval times or simply using anything you regard as a 'good spice.'

IN MORE MODERN ENGLISH

1. Cut the rabbit into pieces and boil them well in the broth.
2. Pare and mince the ginger root.
3. Mix the wine with vinegar, spices, currants and ginger. Stir well and boil.
4. Put the rabbit in the syrup[1], boil, reduce heat, and simmer until tender.
5. Put the rabbit on a serving plate and cover it with currants and the sauce it was boiled in.

[1]This sauce is called in medieval terms, poynaunt, a sweet and sour sauce. Go easy on the amount of sour vinegar and the fresh ginger.

Rabbit in Broth—Connynges in grauey

This is from the 14th century English cookbook *Forme of Cury*

ORIGINAL RECIPE:

Connynges in grauey:

Take connynges: smyte hem to pecys: perboile hem and drawe hem with a gode broth, with almaundes, blaunched and brayed. Do þerinne sugar, and powdour gynger, and boyle it and the flessh þerwith; flour it with sugur & with powdour gynger & serue forth.

INGREDIENTS	
Rabbit	Sugar
Gode broth (made without bread crumbs)[1]	Ginger (powder)
Almonds	

[1] Use any broth you like

DIRECTIONS

1. Cut the rabbit into serving-sized pieces; parboil until done and remove from the water.
2. Put the rabbit pieces in a large pot and cover with any broth you like. Add the ground almonds & spices. Bring to a boil, then reduce heat and simmer for a few minutes.
3. Move the rabbit to a serving dish, pour broth over the rabbit, and sprinkle sugar and ginger on top.
4. Serve forth!

Medieval Rabbit 15th Century—Czech

INGREDIENTS	
MEDIEVAL:	Clove
2 Rabbit legs	Saffron
3/4 cup red wine	2 Onions
3-1/3 cups unsalted beef stock	2 apples
Breadcrumbs	
Pepper	MODERN:
Ginger	To the rest, add 2tbs flour salt sugar

DIRECTIONS — MEDIEVAL

1. Chop onion and apple roughly.
2. Pour red wine into a pot. Add chopped onion and apple.
3. Fill the pot with stock.
4. Bring to a boil, then turn it down, cover, and cook for about an hour, until the meat is tender.
5. When the meat is tender, remove it from the sauce. Strain the sauce. Use a wooden spoon (because there was no plastic in medieval times) to try to push some of the onion and apple through the sieve to add flavor to the sauce.
6. Season the sauce with ginger, cloves, pepper, and saffron.
7. Add breadcrumbs until you have the desired thickness of your sauce.
8. Pour the sauce on a plate. Put a piece of rabbit meat in the center of the sauce and serve with ale (beer will do) and thick, warm bread.

DIRECTIONS – MODERN

1. Chop onion and apples into small cubes.
2. Melt butter in a pan and fry the rabbit in it, seasoning with pepper. When it's done, remove it from the pan.
3. Add the onion and apple into the same pan. Fry until they're slightly brown.
4. Then add wine. When it evaporates, add a tablespoon or so of flour and fry for a minute.
5. Add beef stock and bring it to a boil.
6. Put the meat back into this sauce with the resting juices and saffron.
7. Cover and cook for an hour.
8. Fry the apples in butter, add sugar, ginger and a little water. Cook it about 15 minutes until the apples are melted. Thicken it with breadcrumbs. Mash up the apples if they're still solid.
9. Place this apple puree on a plate, spoon sauce around the side and place a piece of rabbit meat on top.
10. Garnish it with parsley or any sprig of green herb for color.

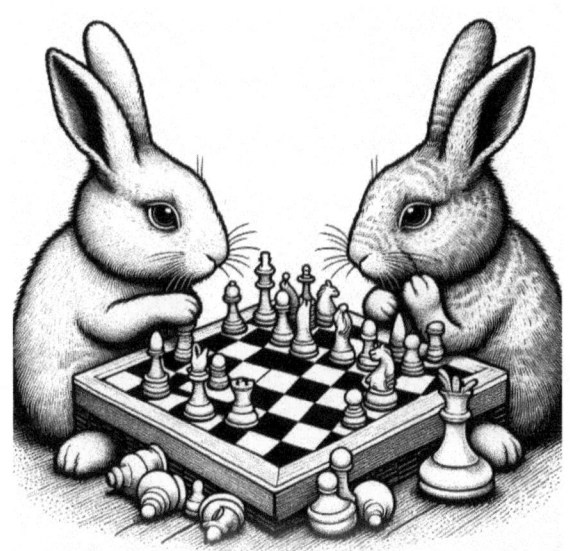

Medieval Rabbit Stew with Spices *Civé de connin*

This recipe is from the late 14th Century's French cookbook Ménagier de Paris, 1393, or *The Good Wife's Guide*. It's a book written by a much older husband for his young wife that includes sections on managing a household, servants and horses, in addition to recipes.

Some historians have said vegetables tasted different in medieval times. This is possible for many reasons. We know from the Chillingham cattle, a herd that has bred only amongst itself for the last 800 years, how different our modern cows are from medieval cattle. Musicologists know music sounds very different today than in medieval times, not merely for different styles but because they had a different concept of tuning and a different tuning system.

We know that the climate and landscape has varied. The battlefield on which Robert the Bruce fought Bannockburn is not what we see there today. There was a Little Ice-Age from around the 1500s to 1800s. All of this would change the quality of the soil, the growing season, and more, which could impact the taste of food grown. So vegetables may well have tasted different then—meaning any medieval recipe we try may not taste like what they tasted. Regardless, it gives us at least a glimpse into the medieval world.

INGREDIENTS

1 rabbit (about 3 pounds)	Ginger
A bit of lard or oil	Cinnamon
Thick sourdough bread	Nutmeg
Wine	Long pepper [2]
Good red wine vinegar	Guinea pepper (grains of paradise)
Good stock	A pinch of ground cloves
2-3 chopped onions	A small pinch of salt
A little bit of verjuice [1]	

[1] substitute white wine vinegar, apple cider vinegar or lemon juice
[2] not a pepper, this actually a very small fruit from a plant grown in India

DIRECTIONS

1. Roast a rabbit on a spit, cut into pieces. Cook the onions. Fry the rabbit and onions. Deglaze with vinegar and reduce just a bit.

2. Grill the bread then soak it with stock and wine. Mix, add the powdered spices that have been diluted with verjuice, add the rest of the verjuice. Mix liquid with rabbit. Cook together for 45 minutes.

3. The Civé should be brown, its richness cut by the vinegar, and it should be moderately salted and seasoned.

Rabbit in Wine or Ale Sauce

This is from the 15th century English cookbook known as *MS Harley 5401*

ORIGINAL
For to make Conys in Hogepoche.

Scald hyr, þan hew hyre in gobets all raw & seth hyr in hyr awne grece, & cast þerto ale or wyne a gode cup full, & mynce onyons small & do þerto, & bole it & serof it forth.

INGREDIENTS:	
Rabbit, whole or in pieces	Ale or red wine
Olive oil, substituting for rabbit grease	Minced onion

DIRECTIONS

1. Scald the rabbit in boiling water; remove and drain well. If using a whole rabbit, cut in pieces.

2. Heat olive oil in a large skillet. Fry the rabbit pieces in the hot oil until browned. Add the minced onion and enough ale or wine to not quite cover the pieces.

3. Bring to a boil, then reduce heat. Simmer until the onion is cooked. Then serve.

Although the recipe doesn't mention spices, add any medieval seasonings: salt, pepper, cubeb, ginger, cinnamon, savory, etc. Or anything you like.

Hogepoche is also spelled as *hochepotte* or *hoggepotte* in other medieval recipes the original meaning of the word implied *shaken* or *stirred*. Not quite the way James Bond put it.

Rabbit with Figs and Mudéjar Spices

Conejo con Higos al Estilo Mudéjar

INGREDIENTS

1-2 tablespoons honey (try rosemary honey)	Sprigs of mint, thyme, and parsley
1/4 cup sherry vinegar	1/4 teaspoon saffron threads, crushed
1-inch piece of fresh ginger, cut in half	1/4 cup hot water
1/4 teaspoon black peppercorns	1/4 olive oil
1/4 teaspoon coriander seeds	1/3 cup blanched almonds
1/4 teaspoon mustard seeds	3 cloves garlic
1/8 teaspoons anise seeds	1 rabbit, 2-1/2 to 3 pounds cut into 8 pieces
1 inch piece of cinnamon	Rabbit liver, cut up, optional
3 cloves	Salt
2 cups water	Ground black pepper
12 dried figs, stems removed	1/2 cup finely chopped onions
1/2 cup white wine	

DIRECTIONS

1. Combine honey, vinegar, ginger, peppercorns, coriander, mustard, aniseeds, cinnamon, and clove in a saucepan with 2 cups water. Bring to a boil and simmer 5 minutes. Remove from heat. Add the sprigs of herbs and figs. Cover and let them soak for at least 2 hours.

2. Crush the saffron in a mortar. Add 1/4 cup of hot water. Steep at least 15 minutes.

3. Heat the oil in a large sauté pan and fry the almonds and garlic until they are lightly golden. Skim them out and set aside.

4. Add the rabbit pieces and liver to the hot oil and saute on medium heat until they are light brown on all sides. Remove the liver pieces. Add the chopped onion and continue sautéing. Put the fried almonds, garlic and liver in a blender with the wine and process to make a smooth paste.

5. Remove the figs from the spiced liquid and set aside. Strain the liquid and reserve it. Discard the spices and herbs. Add 1-1/2 cups of the spice liquid to the rabbit with the saffron. Stir in the almond paste. Season with salt and pepper. Cover and simmer 20 minutes. Add the figs to the rabbit and cook until rabbit is tender, another 15 to 20 minutes

NOTES

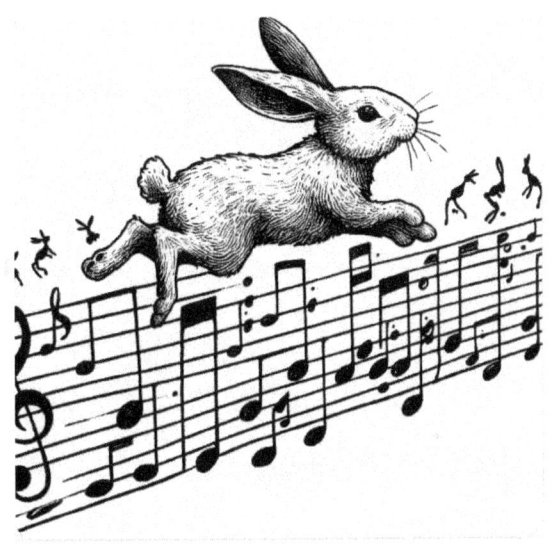

Cooking is both art and experimentation. Be sure to note combinations you try and how you like them and add other recipes you find that you like.

The 'combinations' charts are meant to be used by starting with a base recipe (say Shawn's Fried Rabbit), but roasting instead of frying, and using the spices and seasonings from Rabbit Meatballs with Porcini Tagliatelle and adding any additions you made:

Base Recipe	Cooking Method	Spices	My additions
Shawn's Fried Rabbit	Roasted (Roasted Rabbit in Wine Sauce & Garlic	From Rabbit meatballs in Porcini Tagliatelle	Added chanterelle and morel mushrooms & garlic

Combinations

Base Recipe	Cooking Method	Spices	My Additions:

Base Recipe	Cooking Method	Spices	My Additions:

Base Recipe	Cooking Method	Spices	My Additions:

Base Recipe	Cooking Method	Spices	My Additions:

Base Recipe	Cooking Method	Spices	My Additions:

Other Recipes

My Recipe:

INGREDIENTS

DIRECTIONS

Cooking with Rabbit

My Recipe::
INGREDIENTS

DIRECTIONS

My Recipe::

INGREDIENTS

DIRECTIONS

My Recipe::

INGREDIENTS

DIRECTIONS

My Recipe::
INGREDIENTS

DIRECTIONS

Cooking with Rabbit

My Recipe::
INGREDIENTS

DIRECTIONS

My Recipe::

INGREDIENTS

DIRECTIONS

THANK YOU!

I hope you've found some wonderful new tastes and been inspired to mix and match and experiment with what *you* like! If you've enjoyed the book please consider leaving a review and giving my pages and channels likes and follows.

Facebook:

@laura.vosika.author, @GabrielsHornPress, @Bksandbrews @GlenmirrilFarms

YouTube:

@gabrielshornpress @booksandbrews @wordsmithsawolfhoundintheg4718

Instagram:

@laura_vosika @glenmirrilfarm @booknbrews

I would especially love it if you photograph any of the rabbit dishes you make and post it at any of my sites.

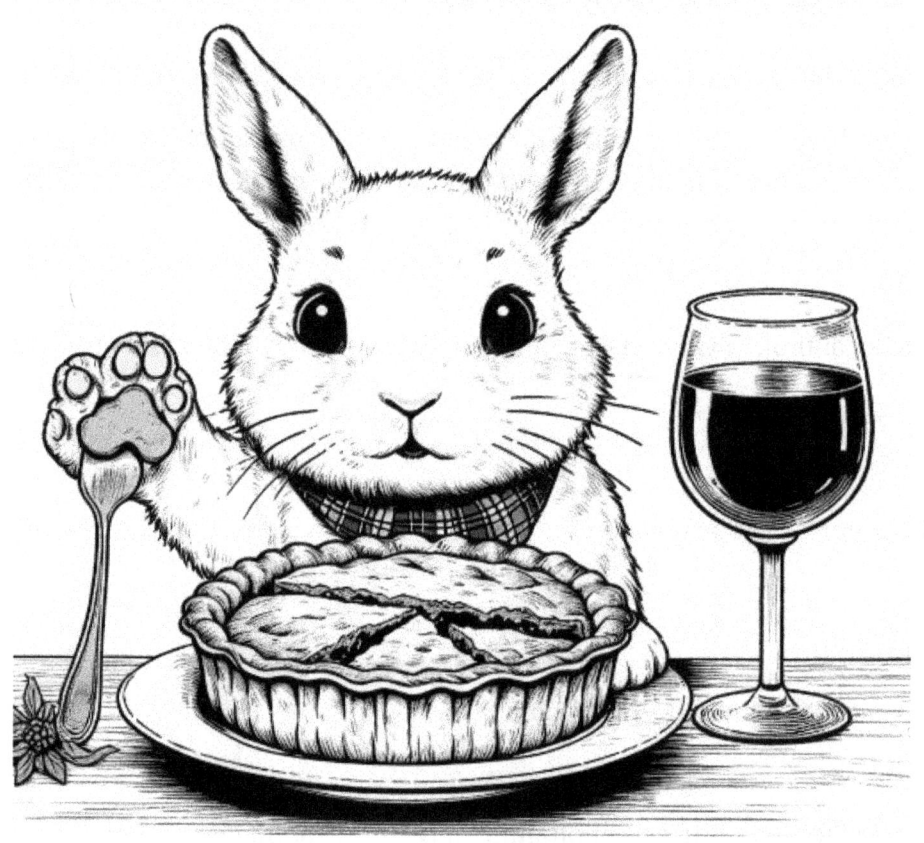

www.ingramcontent.com/pod-product-compliance
Lightning Source LLC
Chambersburg PA
CBHW080441110426
42743CB00016B/3241